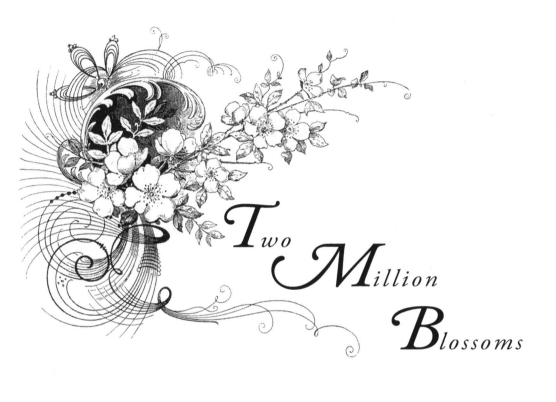

*Two Million Blossoms*

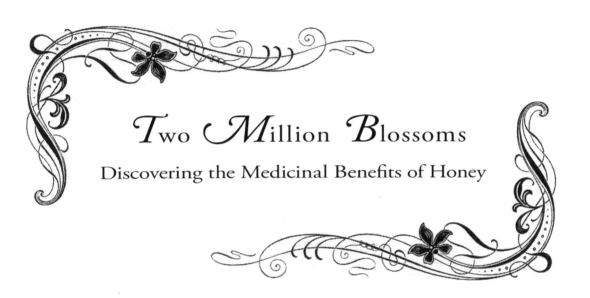

# Two Million Blossoms

## Discovering the Medicinal Benefits of Honey

KIRSTEN S. TRAYNOR, M.S.

**Image Design Publishing**
Middletown, MD

Printed in the United States of America

First Printing, 2011

ISBN  978-0-9723492-1-5

Image Design Publishing
Middletown, MD

www.imagedesignpublishing.com

Edited by Joanne Lane of First Editing

*This book is dedicated to my grandmother Ruth,
whose curiosity and imagination inspired my childhood.*

*And my husband Michael, who has helped me trail the honey bee
through history and around the globe.*

# Contents

**NOTE TO THE READER:**

This book is intended solely as a guide to the medicinal benefits of honey, based on historical research and the published results of laboratory experiments, case studies and clinical trials. The author is not a medical practitioner and thus the book is not intended to be used as a manual for medical self-treatment.

While honey has great therapeutic potential, using honey for medical purposes should only be done under the supervision of your physician. The information presented in this book is intended only as an informational resource. The author assumes no liability and advises that she can not be held responsible for any adverse reactions to honey consumption or applications.

All of the sources used throughout the text are cited in the back of the book. If you desire to use honey, discuss the possibilities with your health care practitioner, who should use the original source material as a guide before deciding on the best possible treatment.

This book is simply intended to acquaint you with the potential medicinal benefits of honey. Seek out appropriate medical help if you have a medical problem and follow the advice of your attending physician.

# *Foreword*

This delightful book Kirsten has written is the book I wanted to write myself twenty years ago, but I never progressed further than producing outlines for the chapters. I felt it was very important the public know about the information I was finding and discovering on the potential of honey, as it could prevent people from suffering needlessly from ailments that detracted from their quality of life. But I was also very aware that more scientific research was needed to be able to persuade the present-day medical profession to seriously consider using honey as a medicine. Research always turns up as many new questions as it does answers, and I am still working on finding the answers, so the book never got written. I was also hesitant to face the difficulty of writing something that the general public would easily understand. It was for these reasons that I was so pleased to be approached for help by someone with the writing ability that I longed for, who had a keen interest in writing such a book, and an excellent understanding of the subject.

Kirsten first contacted me in 2005 when she asked for my permission to put some of my articles on the website she ran as an informational resource for beekeepers and bee product consumers. She was in the process of expanding the section on the medicinal benefits of bee products. In our ongoing correspondence she asked me for copies of additional papers I had written. They helped her gain a better grasp of the medical uses of honey which she was researching for a book for the lay public, as part of her work under a German Chancellor Fellowship from the Alexander von Humboldt Foundation. Further into this project she told me, "I am enjoying the work on my book, learning to find a good balance between describing scientific facts and translating them into interesting, understandable snippets for the lay public. I am trying to explain complicated ideas in a simple and entertaining manner, in hopes of appealing to a larger audience. The goal is to raise awareness for the benefits of hive products among people who have nothing to do with bees." This was good news for me; Kirsten had a BA degree with a major in English and was well qualified to write. I could see from the questions she asked that she also had an excellent ability to understand the science and medicine involved and was taking a rigorous approach to distinguishing facts from myth. My impression that she would do this sort of writing well was confirmed when I was sent a copy of material she had written.

As Kirsten gathered more and more information, she realized that the medicinal benefits of honey had grown into a book length manuscript. She said that she would like to co-write it with me, a proposal to which I enthusiastically agreed. That arrangement worked very well, but as I read through the various chapters that Kirsten sent me to check, I realized that the writing and intellectual input were all hers and my input was solely that of a researcher. There was also a lot of material which Kirsten obtained herself from interviewing clinicians working with honey. Consequently I felt it would not be appropriate for me to be credited as an author and that she should get all the credit. But I am in complete agreement with what she has written.

What Kirsten has written in this book should be distinguished from what is generally written about the health-promoting properties of honey. The many claims that are made, which are not supported by scientific research or medical evidence, add to the widespread prejudice that there is against any medicine that is not the product of the research and advertising of pharmaceutical companies. There is much recycling of misinformation, especially on websites. Kirsten has been very careful to seek and use only information that is based on the findings of scientific research and professional clinical practice.

Readers of this book should find it an interesting and enjoyable learning experience, and very beneficial for their health.

Dr. Peter Molan
Associate Professor of Biochemistry
Director of the Honey Research Unit
Department of Biological Sciences
University of Waikato

# Acknowledgements

Without the help and support of many, *Two Million Blossoms* would never have been written. In 2006, I received the German Chancellor Fellowship from the Alexander von Humboldt (AvH) Foundation. I am grateful for the opportunity afforded by the AvH foundation, which gave me the opportunity to learn as much as I could about bees and beekeeping - a journey that burned through two used cars, as my husband and I traveled over 55,000 miles for 18 months through Western Europe to meet beekeepers, medical doctors and researchers.

I also extend my thanks to Dr. Otto Boecking, my host and mentor during my AvH Fellowship at the Institute for Bee Research in Celle, Germany. Kind, knowledgeable and supportive, Otto gave me the freedom to pursue multiple avenues of research and encouraged me to explore and interact with many researchers. My thanks also to the researchers and staff there that welcomed me and made me feel at home, especially Dr. Werner von der Ohe, head of the institute, the master beekeepers Herr Hansgeorg Schell and Herr Helmut Schönberger, and bee whisperer Herr Guido Eich. I also wish to recognize Frau Kierig, who helped me obtain many research papers, and the remarkable gardener Herr Dubicki, who manages the extensive gardens.

Many individuals helped me from afar, including the courteous head of the International Bee Research Association, Richard Jones. He kindly arranged for me to gain access to the Eva Crane collection, the largest archives of apiary literature, which had recently been transferred to the National Library of Wales in Aberystwyth. The affable Gwyn Tudur Davies, who supervised the acquisition, was still in the process of cataloguing the collection but allowed my husband and me to visit the stacks and select books and manuscripts ourselves.

I am grateful to Dr. Peter Molan, who encouraged me in this project from the very beginning. His research inspired me to write this book and make scientific research available to the public in an understandable format. Not only is Peter incredibly generous with his time, he also invited us to stay in his home when my husband and I visited New Zealand in 2010. He and his wife Alyson share a wonderful sense of humor and remain positive even when life places unexpected hurdles in their path. This book would not have been possible without Peter's decades of hard work uncovering the medicinal uses of honey. Peter Molan—the Man of Manuka—continues to be an inspiration to me and countless others researching honey.

Other people that have given their time generously to answer my questions include:

- Dr. Jost Dustmann, former honey advisor to the German Beekeeping Organization,

- Dr. Arne Simon, oncology specialist at the Bonn Pediatric University Hospital,

- Dr. Jennifer Eddy, family practitioner at Health's Family Medicine Clinic in Eau Claire, Wisconsin,

- Registered nurse Cheryl Dunford, faculty member at Southampton University in the United Kingdom,

- Dr. Nicki Engeseth, food chemist at the University of Illinois,

- Dr. May Berenbaum, phytochemist and head of Entomology at the University of Illinois,

- Dr. Nicola Starkey, animal behavior psychologist at the University of Waikato, New Zealand,

- Dr. Shona Blair, molecular biologist at the University of Sydney,

- Dr. Merle Diamond of the Diamond Headache Clinic in Chicago.

Lastly and most importantly, I would like to thank my husband Michael J. Traynor who is always willing to join me on another adventure. We work together as a team and although I do the writing, he is involved in all aspects of creating and refining our books and articles. I could not ask for a more supportive and helpful husband who continues to inspire me every day. He enabled this book to take shape over the last five years, smoothing rough edges, streamlining content and helping to bring it to market. So even though my name is listed as the author, he deserves equal credit. Together we photographed, designed and created the beautiful images that adorn the book. Thank you Michael for everything.

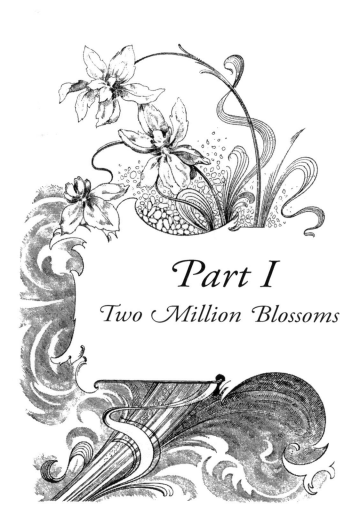

# Part I
## Two Million Blossoms

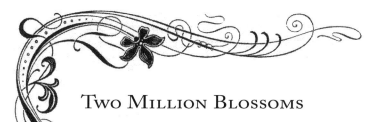

# Two Million Blossoms

*Two million blossoms in a jar.*
*The scent of spring, fresh, sweet*
*with a hint of citrus,*
*spills over your tongue,*
*wafts delicately through your nostrils,*
*as you taste nature's first sweetener—*
*pure, natural, honey.*

- Kirsten S. Traynor

*We* all crave sweets; delicious, sugary, satisfying rewards. Evolution has hardwired our brains to seek out tasty treats. Long before we had a written language, we hunted and searched for our daily food. Observation taught us what we could and couldn't eat. Bitter, rank tastes implied poison while sweet foods screamed at our ravenous prehistoric ancestors, "Eat me, eat me, I'm ripe and safe to swallow!" In the past when provisions were scarce, naturally sweet foods provided the caloric binge our bodies needed to survive.

Mass production of sugar and high fructose corn syrup is a blip on our evolutionary timeline. Our bodies have not had a chance to adapt to the onslaught of cheap sweeteners and rewire our brains. Seeking to avoid the extra calories and still satisfy our sweet tooth, we down artificial sugar-free substitutes and guzzle gallons of diet soda. These artificial sweeteners creep into a vast array of products from salad dressings and yogurts to bread and pickles. But are they good for us? New research has found that artificial sweeteners do not truly satisfy our sweet cravings, causing us to eat more.[1]

Our use of diet sodas has skyrocketed just as the number of obese Americans increased from about 15 percent of the population in the late 1980s to 30 percent in 2000. A quarter-century-long study at the University of Texas Health Science Center at San Antonio tracked weight gain and soda consumption. While at first it appeared that soda in general caused increased weight, a reanalysis of the data showed that only diet soda was the culprit.[2] "On average, for each diet soft drink our participants drank per day, they were 65 percent more likely to become overweight during the next seven to eight years, and 41 percent more likely to become obese,"[3] said Sharon Fowler, M.P.H., from the Health Science Center's department of medicine when she presented her findings at the American Diabetes Association's scientific meeting.

"Millions of people are being exposed to sweet tastes that are not associated with caloric or nutritive consequences."[4] We taste something sweet, but our bodies do not receive the calories the sweet taste normally implies. This may create an imbalance that causes us to underestimate calorie intake and overeat.[5]

Our ancestors found a sweet solution to satisfying our sugar cravings eons ago. A vibrant cave painting hidden in the Cave of the Spider on the banks of the River Cazunta in Valencia, Spain testifies to our ancient infatuation with honey. Painted in bold red paint, an artist captured an androgynous figure trusting his life to three thin grass ropes to rob honey out of a hive high up on a cliff wall. Using a curved dip in the wall to accentuate the cavernous hive, the artist depicted an ancient honey hunting scene, believed to date to 6000 BC.[6] The shadowy figure's long arm ends in a tight grip on a hollowed out gourd or hand woven basket, ready to hold the stolen bounty, as enlarged bees buzz around.

Numerous tribes throughout the world still hunt honey in an almost identical fashion, risking their lives for a delectable reward. While we mostly enjoy honey as an occasional sweetener, our ancestors used honey primarily for medicinal purposes. Hippocrates, the father of modern medicine who lived around 430 BC, used honey extensively for treating rotting wounds and flushing the internal system. The ancient Egyptians bandaged sores with a mixture of honey and oil.

Gathered by tens of thousands of bees from millions of blooming plants, honey contains an impressive array of beneficial properties. Throughout time honey has helped cure a wide range of disorders. Up until World War II doctors wrapped infected tissues of the battle wounded with honey dressings, saving countless limbs from gangrene and amputation. This sweet, mercurial concoction even relieved opposing ailments, alleviating both constipation and diarrhea.

Cultures as far apart as Polynesia, Russia, Sri Lanka and Mexico soothed sore throats with a spoonful of honey. Honey solutions dipped into the eyes prevented cataracts and scarring. Sailors were often fed a ration of honey to prevent scurvy. We think of contraceptives as a fairly modern invention, but our early ancestors used honey as an effective ingredient in an ancient spermicide to avoid unplanned pregnancy.

Sadly with the advent of modern medicine and antibiotics many natural remedies fell out of favor and much of the herbal healing knowledge of ancient doctors was lost. They may not have understood the science of why a particular ingredient worked, but they certainly knew that it produced the desired results.

Long before Sir Alexander Fleming discovered his famous antibiotic penicillin, Egyptian doctors knew particular molds healed wounds. Archeologists have even uncovered antique metal Roman stamps, which were used to press names into blocks of medicines. Some of these stamps contained the Latin word *penicille*, which translates into mold.[7] For a long time researchers disregarded this simple word, for why would doctors used mold as medicine.

Just as the mysteries of penicillin were unraveled in the last century, many of the secrets surrounding honey have recently been laid bare. In the twenty-first century we are coming to the end of the antibiotic age. Multi-resistant bacteria wreak havoc in our operating rooms and hospitals, turning routine care into deadly disasters. Grappling for new solutions in the face of such rapidly evolving pathogens, doctors have rediscovered the healing touch of honey.

Although the medical use of honey is not wide spread in the United States, it is far more common in Europe. From 1984 until 2009, the

French medical doctor Descottes applied honey to 3,012 lesions with excellent results of wound healing.[8]

Honey gauze bandages were approved as a medical device by the Food and Drug Administration (FDA) in 2008 and are currently available by prescription only.[9] Such bandages have been used successfully to treat a wide variety of wounds, including non-responsive diabetic foot ulcers that refused to heal using a variety of standard medical practices like silver dressings.[10,11,12] In Europe, anyone can purchase medical grade honey over the counter in pharmacies.

As scientists examine nature's first sweetener with the machinery of modern medicine, they revive the knowledge of our ancestors. Case studies, laboratory research and clinical trials confirm honey heals many ailments and has revealed surprising new insights:

- Consuming honey instead of sugar reduces weight gain, improves memory and reduces anxiety

- Diabetic ulcers and infected wounds that stagnate under traditional care heal rapidly with honey

- Burn victims and amputees, including civilian casualties during the Iraq war, respond well to honey bandages, making painful skin grafts unnecessary

- A spoonful of honey helps alleviate side effects of head or neck radiation in cancer patients

- Honey proves more effective and safer than children's cough medicines

- Functioning as both a prebiotic and probiotic, honey stimulates intestinal health, eliminates diarrhea and functions as a natural laxative

- Cataracts respond well to stingless bee honey from South America

American researchers often hesitate to investigate the medicinal effects of honey in rigorous medical trials for several reasons, including lack of research funds and the stigma of practicing "folk medicine". In light of mounting biological evidence to support the use of honey in modern wound care and preliminary clinical evidence that demonstrates wound healing benefits, U.S. medical researchers are calling for enlarged clinical trials to confirm its therapeutic effects.[13] With additional funding and support, more scientific discoveries on the medical benefits of honey will surely be uncovered.

Although our predecessors knew honey healed, they were unable to unravel how it worked. With the help of technology and new scientific knowledge, we can start to answer this question, unearthing the elusive temperament of two million blossoms in a jar.

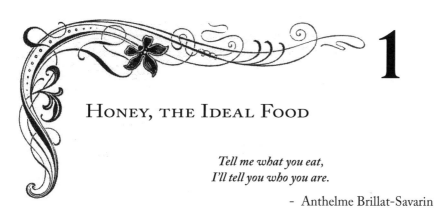

# HONEY, THE IDEAL FOOD

*Tell me what you eat,*
*I'll tell you who you are.*

- Anthelme Brillat-Savarin

*If* you are what you eat, then honey makes you sweet. While many nutritionists believe honey is just a sugar substitute, in truth it affects the body much differently than white table sugar. New studies show that unlike sucrose, long term honey consumption does not lead to weight gain.

If you have never tasted an unheated, unblended honey from a local beekeeper, you are missing a gourmet experience. It dissolves over your tongue in sweet ecstasy. The taste of spring honey liberates aromas of fresh rain and newly opened blossoms. Each hive of honey bees visits a slightly different spread of flowers to sip nectar, which the honey bees struggle to bring home and turn into honey. The lighter the honey is in color, the milder it tends to taste, while darker honeys burst with robust tangs.

9

Modern grocery stores and chain restaurants have taught us to expect the same exact taste each and every time for a given product. To meet this demand for consistency, honey packers blend different honeys to achieve the consumer's ideal. Wine connoisseurs do not expect a particular wine from a vineyard to taste the same from year to year, relishing the nuances imparted by weather and other factors. Yet vintners control exactly what grapes they harvest for a particular wine. Beekeepers can only steer their ladies in the right direction by placing their hives near good nectar sources. They do not control what flowering bounty the bees decide to visit. So let us learn to enjoy the gradations of flavor; the different shades of aromas that tantalize our taste buds when we spoon into nature's first sweetener. Honey, as you will continue to discover in the following pages, is a delicious, healthy, diverse treat that proves, once and for all, that medicine can be sweet.

## SMOTHERED IN SUGAR

Refined table sugar is composed of the complex sugar sucrose. Honey contains mainly the two simple sugars fructose and glucose. The body can immediately assimilate and use glucose, the fuel source that drives almost all bodily functions including the brain. The glucose in honey provides instant energy. To utilize the fructose, the body must first convert it to glucose, making this second type of sugar a slow release form of energy.

But what exactly is honey and why do the bees make it? To survive the winter, honey bees do not hibernate. Instead, a colony clusters tightly together inside their hive, forming a close-knit ball of quivering bees. The female worker bees continually flex their wing muscles without flapping their wings. This movement generates heat that protects the colony and the single queen hidden in the center of the cluster. As the bees on the edge start to chill, they crawl into the center of the ball. To generate this heat, the bees need a food source. The honey provides the bees with a carbohydrate energy source during the winter dearth of nectar.

To make one pound of honey, bees must visit over two million blossoms. A single female worker bee will only make 1/12th of a teaspoon of honey in her lifetime. If you added up the total distance flown to make a single pound of honey, the bees involved would have circumnavigated the globe three times.

## THE MORAL OF THE MYTH

According to a Greek myth, Cronus had learned that one of his children would kill him and take over as ruler of the gods. To avoid the prophecy he devoured his offspring each time his wife Rhea bore a child. Frustrated by her husband's murderous ways, Rhea fled to the island of Crete to deliver her sixth child Zeus. She then tricked her husband by handing over a stone wrapped in swaddling cloth, which Cronus quickly swallowed whole.

Hidden away on the island of Crete in a cave on Mount Dicte, the newborn Zeus ate honey from the sacred bee Melissa and drank milk from the goat Amaltheia. Guarded by armed men, who clashed their swords against their armor each time the young child cried out, Zeus grew strong on this special diet of milk and honey. As a young man, he fulfilled the prophecy, slaying his father and freeing his five swallowed siblings.[1]

The association between milk and honey survives to this day in numerous cultures. Even in the United States, a common folk remedy for a child who can not fall asleep is a glass of warm milk with honey. Ancient cultures prized honey harvested from wild hives, using the delicacy primarily for medicinal purposes.

While other countries still consume honey in greater quantities, it has sadly fallen out of favor in the United States. Easily dispensed from any container, dry, granulated sugar has relegated honey to occasional use in a cup of tea. According to the U.S. Department of Agriculture (USDA) Economic Research Service, the average American consumed over 66 lbs of sugar and 48 lbs of corn syrup in 2010, while they enjoyed just one pound of honey.[2] The consumption of sugar and high fructose corn syrup continues to climb, as obesity rates skyrocket. The USDA, Center for Nutrition Policy and Promotion noted a much higher rate of sugar consumption: Americans consume a whopping 158 lbs per year.[3] That's over three pounds per week.

So what exactly are we pouring into our bodies at such an alarming rate? Table sugar is pure sucrose, a complex (disaccharide) sugar produced from sugar cane or sugar beets. To obtain sugar's pure white color, manufacturers purify raw cane sugar with phosphoric acid or filter it, before running it through a bed of activated carbon or bone char. Table sugar provides the body with empty calories and no other nutrients or benefits. Before the body can use the energy in sugar, it must first convert the complex sugar into simple sugars.

The explosion of high fructose corn syrup as an ingredient in everyday food has mimicked the climb in obesity rates. Many believe high fructose corn syrup is the culprit behind escalating numbers of diabetics.

Yet there is no evidence to suggest high fructose corn syrup is worse than table sugar.[4,5] High consumption of both has been conclusively linked to weight gain and myriad ailments that coincide with flabbiness, such as increased risk of heart disease, diabetes, and elevated blood pressure.[6] The excess sugar is converted into fat, which over time adds surplus pounds.

In comparison, the body easily absorbs the main components of natural honey, the simple sugars glucose and fructose. In addition, honey also delivers trace amounts of enzymes, vitamins, minerals, organic acids, amino acids, hormones, bioflavonoids, antioxidants, aromatic substances, and water. See the "Components of Honey" table for a complete list.

Although the content is minor, honey contains up to 18 of the 20 essential amino acids; a surprising diversity. As doctors can testify, minute quantities can still have a large impact on our general health. The types of amino acids vary from one floral source to the next.

The predominant acid in honey is gluconic acid. As far back as 1975, researchers in France showed consumption of gluconic acid increased calcium absorption.[7] Rates of osteoporosis continue to climb in the United States, especially among women. According to the National Osteoporosis Foundation, 10 million Americans suffer from osteoporosis.[8] Of those 10 million, 80 percent are women. An additional 34 million individuals have low bone mass, meaning they are at risk of developing this disabling disease. Anything that helps us to naturally absorb calcium and retain our bone mass is worth noting.

In a long term animal study carried out in New Zealand, researchers found that honey fed animals showed a slight but significant increase in bone density compared to animals fed a diet that contained table sugar or a sugar-free substitute.[9] If the same proves true in humans, honey could help us retain our bone mass as we age.

Organic acids also chelate heavy metals, which removes them from the bloodstream. They thus can "synergistically enhance the action of other antioxidants, such as phenolics".[10] Honey contains enzymatic and non-enzymatic antioxidants, which are described in greater detail below.

Sweeter than sugar, honey provides a greater sensation of sweetness with fewer calories. According to German health nutritionist Renate Frank, a tablespoon of honey provides the equivalent sweetness of nine sugar cubes, but contains only the calories of five.[11] While it is easy to plow through a large chocolate bar or a cup of ice cream, you would be hard pressed to consume the same weight in honey. After a few small spoonfuls, honey satisfies your sweet craving and leaves you feeling full.

Honey increases the natural sweetness of other ingredients, while reducing the perceived sourness. It also minimizes "the bitterness intensity and increases the acceptability of savory products by modifying saltiness perception".[12] In short, honey positively enhances culinary experiences and diminishes those we typically find distasteful.

## COMPONENTS OF HONEY

| Carbohydrates | Enzymes | Vitamins | Minerals | Organic acids | Hormones | Aromatic substances |
|---|---|---|---|---|---|---|
| *Simple Sugars:* Fructose Glucose | Glucose oxidase Phosphatase Invertase Diastase Catalase | Vitamin C Vitamin B Vitamin $B_2$ Vitamin $B_6$ Vitamin H Riboflavin Niacin Pantothenic acid Folate | Calcium Phosphorus Sodium Potassium Iron Zinc Magnesium Selenium Copper Manganese Sulphur Chromium | Gluconic acid Citric acid Lactic acid Acetic acid Formic acid Malic acid | Acetylcholine | Carbon acids Esters |
| *Disaccharides:* Maltose Sucrose | | | | | | |

### ACCESSIBLE ANTIOXIDANTS

While the word phytochemical may sound complex, it breaks down into "phyto" meaning plant and "chemical". Phytochemicals are nutrients derived from plants that actively promote human health, either protecting against or preventing the development of different diseases.

Plants churn out these chemicals to protect themselves. In addition to animals, microbes and fungi feed on plants, so to avoid becoming lunch, plants exude chemicals that guard against these insidious attacks. Some of these plant produced chemicals convey beneficial effects when consumed, defending us against the onset of disease.

Phytochemicals have been discovered in honey, which should come as no surprise, since honey is derived from plant nectar. One would expect that beneficial properties of specific plants might very well exist in the nectar it produced, which bees then convert into honey. Most phytochemicals have antioxidant properties. These safeguard our cells from oxidative damage, which in turn diminishes our risk of developing cancer and other ailments.

"Honey is known to be rich in both enzymatic and non-enzymatic antioxidants, including catalase, ascorbic acid (vitamin C), flavonoids and alkaloids."[13] We bandy about the term antioxidant on a regular basis. Media reports abound that state antioxidants are good for us. But what exactly do they do? Antioxidants help stabilize or deactivate dangerous atoms called free radicals, before the little guys have a chance to attack healthy cells.

Which leads us to the question of what constitutes a free radical? Free radicals are atoms or small group of atoms with an odd number of electrons. Electrons like to exist in pairs. Through oxidation, an atom can either be missing an electron or have an extra, making them extremely unstable. These unbalanced free radicals hunt around for an extra electron, ripping them out of healthy atoms. In a dangerous domino effect, these now destabilized atoms must filch a new electron to regain their equilibrium.

When free radicals steal an electron from important cellular elements such as DNA, or damage protective cell membranes, they unleash potential problems that can escalate into cancer and other medical disorders including "heart disease, stroke, cataracts, Alzheimer's, arthritis and some symptoms of old age".[14]

Oxidants form naturally when we breathe (normal aerobic respiration) and during metabolism and inflammation, but external stress factors such as alcohol, smoking, sunlight, and pollution increase the production of free radicals. Our entire cellular make-up undergoes a process of oxidation as we age - a natural deterioration process. One researcher described oxidative damage quite graphically: "Our bodies are going rancid."[15] Much like rust wears down a machine, free radicals degrade our health over time.

The consumption of antioxidants can help protect against this deterioration by slowing down oxidation. Honey bolsters our body in its fight against everyday stresses by providing it with as many antioxidants as fresh fruit or vegetables. The level of antioxidants varies from one type of honey to the next. We all know that brown rice, swaddled in a nutrient and fiber rich hull, provides better nutrition than white rice. Whole wheat bread supplies the body with more vitamins than the empty calories of white bread.

The same is true of honey. Darker honeys, in general, have greater quantities of antioxidants.[16] When testing the antioxidant level of 14 different varietal honeys, biochemists discovered buckwheat honey from Illinois had the highest level.[17] Buckwheat honey harvested in other regions also rated highly in antioxidant levels. Dark, almost black buckwheat honey tastes very different from the clover honey most Americans know. Its stout, robust flavor contains overtones of licorice and malt. Light, lemony black locust or acacia honey contained the lowest levels of antioxidants. Yet even black locust honey had three times the antioxidants of a substitute honey solution mixed from fructose, glucose, maltose and water.

## Save me Some Soy Beans

Beekeepers move honey bee hives into endless acres of soy beans to pollinate the crop. The honey the bees make from the inconspicuous flowers consistently has high levels of antioxidants.[18] Unfortunately for consumers, most beekeepers market soy bean honey as wildflower. Beekeepers have not yet had the courage to proudly proclaim "Soybean Honey" on their label, said Dr. Nicki Engeseth, a food chemist with the Department of Food Science and Human Nutrition at the University of Illinois. Perhaps they fear silly questions like, "Will soy bean honey give me gas?" She hopes this may change in the future, since this variety of honey is such a reliable source of antioxidants.[19]

## Honey Saves Food From Spoilage

Dr. Engeseth, an expert in antioxidants and oxidation, has studied honey's beneficial effects on food products like meat. Foods we consume are prone to oxidation. As the fats—what scientists call lipids—start to break down, food turns rancid. Honey protects the lipids, helping to preserve foods.

Most people simply do not realize they are eating foods that have started to go rancid, Dr. Engeseth explained during an interview. "These products pose a health risk," Dr. Engeseth said. "They are loaded with free radicals. If you keep a previously opened bottle of vegetable oil in your cupboard, after a few months it will smell like paint when you open it."

We don't think twice about keeping a bottle of vegetable oil for several months or years. "Oxidation strongly changes the taste and odor of the food," Dr. Engeseth said. In her experience, most people have adapted to these off flavors as we are so used to eating oxidized foods we can't taste the difference anymore.

For some of her experiments she needed freshly sliced deli meat. The clerk servicing the deli counter ensured her the meat had been cut that morning, but she insisted he slice some fresh as she waited. "Even when we store thinly sliced meats in the refrigerator, we can detect oxidation within six hours."[20] Honey stops the browning of fruits and vegetables and the oxidation of meats, keeping them fresh and safe to eat longer.[21]

The ancient Egyptians and Romans were aware of honey's protective qualities long before modern research rediscovered this fact. Lacking refrigeration, the Egyptians used vats of honey to preserve their meat.

Dr. Engeseth doesn't know how much oxidized food a person must consume to raise their risk of developing cancer, but diets high in heavily oxidized foods have been conclusively linked to greater cancer incidence. Some foods, especially fried foods, contain mutagens; these have adverse effects on genetic material, potentially leading to the development of tumors and cancer. Antioxidants in honey have revealed antimutagenic properties, which counteract the negative effects of mutagens.[22]

## THE SKINNY ON BAD CHOLESTEROL

Bad cholesterol, properly known as low density lipoprotein (LDL) cholesterol, is also prone to oxidation. Oxidation modifies these nasty culprits; once oxidized, LDL cholesterol causes plaque build-up in the arteries. Too much plaque hardens the arteries, which can eventually lead to heart attacks and strokes.[23] In lab tests, honey displayed the ability to significantly reduce oxidation of LDLs.[24]

While this does not automatically mean honey will have the same protective effect in humans, the possibility does exist. In a small clinical trial, Dr. Engeseth and colleagues had 25 healthy human subjects consume five different hot beverages on separate occasions.[25] The series of drinks included 1) water, 2) buckwheat honey in water, 3) black tea, 4) black tea with buckwheat honey and 5) a sugar mixture that mimicked honey. Only the four tablespoons of buckwheat honey in approximately 16 ounces of water led to a significant increase in the antioxidant capacity of the participant's blood.

According to Dr. Engeseth, the blood of healthy individuals acts as a buffer so the blood is not prone to reflecting changes from the one time consumption of a particular food. Buckwheat honey has a significantly lower antioxidant content than black tea. Yet the antioxidants in buckwheat honey were more readily absorbed by the body, increasing blood antioxidant levels by seven percent.

Dr. Engeseth believes the buckwheat honey jump kicked blood antioxidant levels, because the antioxidant phenolics in honey are present in a different form than those in black tea. When ingested, the antioxidants in honey pass through the internal barrier of the gut with greater ease and so are more accessible to the body.

## REINING IN THE RADICALS

"Excess free radicals are implicated in an ever-growing number of disease conditions, including cancer, cardiovascular diseases and neurodegenerative diseases."[26] Honey, with its readily absorbed antioxidants, could mitigate the impact of free radicals.

According to Dr. Engeseth, "honey may potentially impart significant health benefits to consumers in addition to stabilizing food products."[27] With its high antioxidant content, trace minerals, vitamins and enzymes it is certainly better for you than the empty calories of refined table sugar. Honey could potentially prevent hardening of the arteries linked to heart attacks, making it an ideal ingredient for a heart healthy lifestyle.

## HONEY FLAVONOIDS: TRACES OF PROPOLIS

Honey contains two unique flavonoids called pinocembrin[28] and pinobanksin.[29] These potent antioxidants also exist in much higher concentrations in propolis, another bee product. The colloquial name for propolis is Russian penicillin, because of the frequent use to treat a wide variety of ailments in that country. The bees use this sticky material in the hive to fill cracks. They run a bead of this antifungal, antibacterial and antiviral material along the front entrance of the hive, much like a doormat, to reduce infectious outbreaks. Scientists continue to analyze pinocembrin, as it shows potential for reducing cancer and cognitive brain damage.

# *Interlude*

## *Food Preservation*

Because honey is anti-bacterial and rich in antioxidants, it makes an excellent preservative. As previously stated, the Egyptians used vats of honey to preserve their meat, as noted in the cookbook attributed to Marcus Gavius Apicius, the notoriously greedy Roman gourmand, who was obsessed with the finest quality of food. His lavish feasts made history in the first century AD, earning him ridicule for his obsessive quest of perfection. He detailed the practice of preserving with honey:

> *How to keep meat fresh as long as you like without pickling. Cover meat that you wish to keep fresh with honey, but suspend the receptacle, and use when required. This is better in winter; in summer it will keep in this manner only a few days. You can use this method also with cooked meat.[1]*

When Apicius learned that he no longer had the funds to live the high life, he poisoned his last draught of wine and committed suicide, so appalled was he at the idea of eating the food of the common man.[2]

The style of Apicius' Roman cookbook suggests it was in fact not written by one man. Rather the book is a compilation of recipes, collected over time by generations of cooks, and then named after the notorious gourmand. In the words of chef Sally Grainger:

> *When I read these recipes as a chef, I don't sense the presence of a gourmet reclining at dinner and smelling rose petals and aromatic incense. I smell the damp soot and spices of a working kitchen. I hear the clatter and noise of chopping blocks and the hiss of boiling pots. I imagine an earlier version of this book sitting on a wooden bench*

19

*covered in sooty fingerprints. I imagine some of the current recipes pushed into that copy as loose leaves, others scribbled in the margins in culinary shorthand, the whole thing crying out to be recopied by a secretarial scribe, with no culinary skills, in the format we now have.[3]*

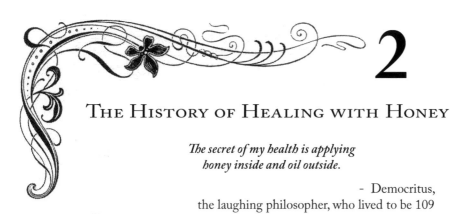

# 2

## The History of Healing with Honey

*The secret of my health is applying*
*honey inside and oil outside.*

- Democritus,
the laughing philosopher, who lived to be 109

$O$ur love affair with honey is an ancient infatuation, recorded in numerous cave paintings and rock art. The world's first sweetener, honey was once worth its weight in gold. Honey and swarms of bees were often the territory of medicine men, used to activate their potency in order to cure disease.[1] Most honey hunters in the past—and indeed today also—were men. In many tribal cultures women were prohibited from interaction with bees for fear their menstrual cycle might contaminate the bees.

In prehistoric times women were not always excluded from this dangerous yet thrilling work. Early inhabitants illustrated the walls of Zombepata Cave, a granite shelter perched high above a tributary of the Mpinge River in Zimbabwe on a farm called Chiconyora - which means

21

'Happy ne'er do well'. The site overlooks a fertile plain and can only be reached after a strenuous climb. One wrong step plunges one down the sheer 180 foot drop to the valley below. Inside early artists decorated the entire length of the wall with a giant frieze painted in red, yellow, purple, black and white pigments ground from minerals near the site. Bees dart in an out of complex patterns, including some which are believed to be bark beehives.[2] A female honey hunter with ample breasts and buttocks carries a long stick to rob honey from giant combs which dwarf her diminutive size in this extraordinary example of prehistoric rock art.[3] Dating is difficult, as the cave had numerous inhabitants starting approximately 35,000 BC; the paintings are believed to be from the late Stone Age.

Another painting discovered in Zimbabwe in a cave used since 8000 BC shows a honey hunter smoking bees to rob honey from the feral hive.[4] The large honey combs dwarf the hunter, demonstrating our ancestors' high regard for honey.

The delicacies from a honey hunt provided our ancestors with carbohydrate rich honey and protein rich bee brood, consumed as a delicacy in many cultures. As bees tend to build their hives in difficult to reach locations, high up in rock crevices or tree hollows, it required great skill and dexterity to harvest the bounty. Small bands of agile hunters typically worked together to do so.

Early artists recorded the thrill of a hunt in Barranc Fondo, Valencia, Spain. Five adventurous hunters climb a ladder; one loses his grip and flails out from the ladder, only one foot still entwined. Twelve individuals wait on the ground below, eager to share in the harvest. The bees constructed their hive onto branches or into a stone crevice, which appears as a dark mass seen from below. Giant, stylized bees take to the air near the nest.

While we enjoy honey for its taste today, we rarely consumed honey as a sweetener in our early history. Our ancestors discovered the healing properties of materials through trial and error. By the time civilizations appeared around 6,000 years ago, mankind had concocted numerous effective topical wound treatments.[5] When early people harvested honey, they used it primarily for medicinal and religious purposes. Through time honey healed infected wounds, softened skin, cured constipation and even made an effective spermicide.

An illness could render the strong and healthy helpless within hours. Without pharmacies, early people depended on the knowledge of healing herbs, roots, animal products and minerals. Honey, animal fat and butter served crucial roles in primitive medicine. Familiarity with the medicinal values of nature's bounty built up over generations and passed from one medicine man or shaman to the next. As protector of the tribe's health, medicine men often enjoyed special status within their community.[6]

## SUMERIAN TABLET

All early cultures with access to honey used it for medicinal purposes. Sometime between 2158 and 2008 BC, during the Third Dynasty of Ur,[7] an unknown Sumerian physician fashioned a small tablet out of moist clay, sharpened a reed stylus to a wedge-shaped edge, and wrote the oldest medical manuscript - fifteen prescriptions in one of the earliest forms of a written language, cuneiform script.[8]

A single written prescription in folk medicine implies a long oral tradition passed from one healer to the next. The Sumerians called the southern part of Mesopotamia home; what is now southeastern Iraq. For over 4,000 years the tablet lay buried in the ruins of Nippur, the religious center of the Sumerians in the Euphrates valley, until it was excavated by an American expedition. The tablet then lay in obscurity, buried in a collection of debris removed from the excavation site for another fifty years, until Dr. Samuel Noah Kramer unearthed it in a collection of the University Museum in Philadelphia.[9]

The red clay tablet, most likely dug from the silt of the Euphrates River, almost succumbed to the burrowing of a worm. Buried for centuries in semi-damp soil, the tablet became soft, inviting the first 'bookworms' to tunnel through. But this particular worm seems to have had an appreciation for writing, since his winding passage only trespassed through an unwritten section of the tablet.[10]

Twelve of the fifteen prescriptions are intended for external use. The very first surviving prescription states:

> Pulverize ...river clay; knead it with water [and] honey; let sea oil and hot cedar oil be spread over it.[11]

Most likely, healers applied this mixture as an external salve for a skin infection or ulcer, forming a mud plaster to protect the wound. Although the author did not include the diseases to be treated, nor mentioned the proportions of ingredients—perhaps guarding the exact recipes so others could not imitate his potent salves—the text confirms Sumerian pharmacology had made significant strides.

A highly developed civilization that created intricate irrigation systems to farm their large agrarian plots, the Sumerians placed great value on honey. One refrain from a Sumerian love song "great is your beauty, sweet as honey"[12] emphasizes the high regard for this delicacy.

## BATTLE WOUNDS AND THE EDWIN SMITH PAPYRUS

Honey was the most commonly used medicament of ancient Egypt, appearing over 500 times in 900 prescriptions for myriad ailments.[13] Egyptian doctors were skilled surgeons who often dealt with trauma and severe wounds. The Edwin Smith Surgical Papyrus—purchased by the American archeologist of the same name on January 20th in 1862 from one Mustapha Aga—details how to handle 48 different types of battle wounds. Sometime during the 19th century the fifteen foot long scroll was chopped into 17 columns.

Edwin Smith desired to translate the papyrus, but he sadly died in 1906 before accomplishing the task. At the time of his death not much of the Egyptian language had been deciphered. Without any bilingual text to help unlock the hieroglyphic code, progress crept along. The key to translating Egyptian hieroglyphs came in the form of the Rosetta Stone, discovered by Napoleon and his troops during their invasion of the Ottoman Empire from 1798-1801.

Instead of the fleur-de-lis, the traditional symbol of France's kings, Napoleon assumed the emblem of the honey bee, a hieroglyphic symbol believed at the time to mean ruler. The industrious insect adorned both his sword and his tunic. A troupe of 151 scientists, scholars and artists accompanied Napoleon's invading force with the sole purpose of recording the cultural heritage, political state and natural history of Egypt.[14]

While demolishing a wall to build the foundation of a fortification, Napoleon's engineers discovered the famous Rosetta Stone; an irregularly shaped granite slab weighing 762 kg (1676 lbs). Inscribed with three versions of the same text—fourteen lines of hieroglyphs, fifty-three lines of Greek and thirty-two lines of what was later discovered to be demotic text—the Stone set off a fierce competition to crack the code. The main contestants were two Egyptologists: the British-born Thomas 'Phenomenon' Young, a polymathic genius and the precocious, brilliant young French linguist Jean-François Champollion.[15] The battle to decipher the Stone lasted two decades, with many other scholars contributing as well.

Another fifty years passed before the hieratic script—a cursive form of the Egyptian hieroglyphics used in the Edwin Smith Papyrus—was translated. The cursive form was typical of everyday writing and is written and read from right to left. When Edwin Smith died in 1906, his daughter donated the papyrus to the New York Historical Society, where it languished until 1920. The society then entrusted the precious papyrus to renowned Egyptologist James Henry Breasted. He devoted himself to its translation for the next ten years, publishing a two-volume English rendition with commentary and medical notes.[16]

Written with a reed pen on papyrus circa 1650-1550 BC—a period haunted by brutal wars—the text featured specific treatments for 48 types of battle wounds sustained during combat. The scribe highlighted every new case and important details of care in red ink, ground from ochre, then switched to black for the body of the text.

Due to the use of hieroglyphics more commonly implmented around 3,000-2,500 BC, James Henry Breasted believed the papyrus was copied from a much older text. He surmised the author of the original text may have been the Egyptian physician Imhotep, who served under the Third Dynasty of the pharaoh Djoser.[17] The author was clearly familiar with treating serious wounds of patients and referred to as a *swnw* (perhaps pronounced soo-noo); the ancient word for physician in the land of the pharaohs.

Each case began with an introductory heading followed by significant symptoms, diagnosis and recommended treatment. The order of the cases followed the flow of the human body, starting with head injuries and proceeding downward. Unfortunately the scribe stopped in the middle of a sentence about treating a pulled vertebra, never completing the treatise.

After listing the key diagnostic features of a specific case, the ancient Egyptian surgeon asserted one of three verdicts on the patient's probable outcome:

> 1) *"a medical condition I can treat"*;
> 2) *"a medical condition I can contend with"*;
> 3) *"a medical condition you will not be able to treat".*[18]

The first statement implies a condition that should respond well to medical care; the second suggests a difficult case that may be surmountable and the physician declares himself willing to try; the third indicates an injury beyond repair, but the patient will still receive help to ease his suffering.

Frequently treatment involved the application of fresh meat, which contained enzymes that aided in the cleansing of wounds, followed by honey bandages changed daily and rest for recuperation.

Nose injuries occurred commonly and received sophisticated care. A *'Break in the column of his nose'* described a case of a broken nose bridge that caused swelling and blood discharge from the nostrils. The surgeon recommended the following treatment:

> *Thou shouldst cleanse* (it) *for him with two plugs of linen saturated with grease in the inside of his two nostrils. Thou shouldst put him at his mooring stakes until the swelling is reduced* (lit. drawn out). *Thou shouldst apply for him stiff rolls of linen by which his nose is held fast. Thou shouldst treat him afterwards with grease, honey and lint, every day until he recovers.* (Edwin Smith Papyrus, Case 11; 510-15)

We will never know exactly what type of grease, *mrht*, the text called for. It could have been anything from vegetable oil to animal fat.[19]

The Egyptian terms for lint vary and were most likely made of plant fiber. The surgeon thus recommended cleansing the nose with oil using a smaller and softer type of linen. Splints to support the broken nose bridge as it heals were made from stiff linen rolled into posts.[20] Lint bandages of oil mixed with honey were applied daily until the nose recovered completely. "Put him at his mooring stakes" meant the patient should be given bed rest.

---

**The Edwin Smith Papyrus**

Unroll and read the Edwin Smith Papyrus at the U.S. National Library of Medicine's Turning the Pages project. Interact with an authentic recreation of the famous surgical text.

http://archive.nlm.nih.gov/proj/ttp/intro.htm

---

Most of the other cases featured in the Edwin Smith Papyrus also received honey and oil bandages to speed recovery, including a lip wound, gaping throat wound, torn ear, perforation to the temple, fractured cheekbone, various cheek wounds, and gaping chest wounds. Other wounds that involved broken or fractured bones, including a dislocated jawbone, fractured collarbone, broken arm, pulled or dislocated rib, were first treated with alum, followed by daily honey treatments.

In many ancient prescriptions, the author lists a host of substitutes for an ingredient, often reinforced with comments like "good, good" or "really proven"; a common practice with drugs that failed to work. But the combination of lint, grease, and honey is recommended for 22 of the 48 prescriptions without any substitutes suggesting the author knew it really worked and nothing else would do.[21]

## Egyptian Medicine And the Ebers Papyrus

The famous Ebers papyrus, found between the legs of a mummy in the Assassif area of the Theban necropolis on the west bank of the Nile River opposite from Luxor, gives a glimpse into traditional Egyptian healing.[22] Written during the reign of Amenhotep I, the papyrus dates to approximately 1550 BC. Carefully set down onto 60 feet of scroll in a clear hand, the papyrus is the longest Egyptian medical text ever recovered - a somewhat haphazard compilation of medical texts numbered by the original scribe. The papyrus is believed to have come from the tomb of a doctor.

Of the many healing prescriptions in the Ebers papyrus, 147 of the recipes for external application contained the ingredient honey.[23] These included dressings to treat wounds, burns, sores, and poor skin conditions due to scurvy. Patients suffering from joint stiffness or after surgery, including circumcision, received topical honey treatments.

> **Honey and Egyptian Medicne**
>
> Honey was a key ingredient in ancient Egyptian medical remedies, appearing in hundreds of prescriptions in the famous medical text the Ebers Papyrus.

The Egyptians didn't just rob honey from feral hives. They housed and managed bee colonies in clay pots, ensuring regular harvests. To increase their honey harvests, the Egyptians exploited the Nile River. They loaded their ceramic hives on flat barges and followed the bloom from warmer to cooler climates. Each region unfurled its blossoms in turn, so the Egyptians harvested honey from the same floral source for an extended period.

Modern day beekeepers mimic their predecessors, transporting thousands of hives each year in large caravans of tractor-trailers up and down both coasts of the United States. Instead of taking advantage of an extended nectar flow, these modern day beekeepers and the millions of bees they truck around, ensure high quality crops of almonds, apples, citrus, and over 90 other fruits and vegetables by providing pollination.

During the reign of the Egyptian pharaohs, honey was valued as highly as gold. To appease the gods, one mighty pharaoh poured fifteen tons of honey into the Nile. Hoping for a sweet afterlife, pharaohs often surrounded themselves in their tombs with honey stores sealed by wax. Since honey stored in airtight containers never spoils, the honey found during the excavation of King Tut's tomb was still edible, despite its long sojourn beneath the sands.

Honey even formed the basis of an Egyptian marriage contract: "I take thee to wife ... and promise to deliver to thee yearly twelve jars of honey."[24] With a jar of honey for every month, let us hope her marriage was as sweet.

A precious commodity, the Egyptians used honey predominantly to appease the gods or treat medical ailments.

An ear remedy, the only recipe to give proportions for the salve, called for: "lint, grease 2/3, honey 1/3, apply to it many times".[25] A modern day equivalent mixed from butter and honey makes a salve of pleasant consistency.

Mixed with oil, honey soothed an upset stomach:

> *You shall than make for him a remedy against it: haematite* (a mineral form of red iron oxide, ground up)*, desh* (unknown term) *and carob, cook in oil and honey; to be eaten by a man at four dawns.* (Ebers 197)

Halitosis—bad breath—seems to have plagued the Egyptians as well. The Ebers papyrus recommends prescriptions to deal with the "illness of the tongue", including a mouthwash of incense, cumin, yellow ochre and honey.[26] (Ebers 700)

Honey even slipped into the treatment regime of gynecological disorders and was included as an ingredient in contraceptives placed in the vagina:

> *To allow a woman to cease conceiving for one year, two years, or three years: qaa part of acacia, carob, dates; grind with henu of honey* (450 ml)*, lint is moistened therewith and placed in her flesh.* (Ebers 783)

This recipe works twofold; first, it mimics the effects of the modern sponge and diaphragm. Second, acacia, when combined with the sugars of honey and dates, ferments into lactic acid,[27] a spermicide still used today as the main component in many contraceptive jellies.

## CONTRACEPTIVES AND THE KAHUN GYNECOLOGICAL PAPYRUS

The oldest Egyptian medical text, the Kahun gynecological papyrus, was discovered with a date recorded on the back, the 29th year of the reign of Amenemhat, believed to have occurred around 1825 BC.[28] Found by Flinders Petrie in 1889 in a town-site excavation near Lahun in Fayum, the settlement thrived during the reigns of Amenemhat and his successors. Consulted so frequently that the papyrus sustained a tear, the ancient owner repaired it with a patch from an administrative scroll.[29]

Although reassembled from many fragments, the Kahun Gynecological papyrus attests to early female medicine and health in the land of the pharaohs. It is ordered very logically with a brief description of symptoms, followed by advice on how to address the patient and summed up with a recommended treatment.

The papyrus contains the first description of a pessary; a suppository inserted into the vagina to prevent conception. Recommended contraceptive ingredients included sour milk;[30] known for its high lactic acid content. Then follows the advice:

> *Honey, sprinkle over her womb, this is to be done on a natron bed.[31]*

The Egyptians used natron, a carbonate salt, as a supreme cleansing agent. The text advocates a mixture of honey and natron which may have proved very effective as a spermicide; natron being an astringent and salt lethal to sperm.

The dark, definitive lines of Kohl and blue-green make-up outlining and emphasizing the eye are inextricably linked with ancient Egypt. Even the poor decorated their eyes. Not only did the makeup beautify and draw attention to the eye, the minerals used had medicinal properties that protected against glare, flies, and disease.[32] Every woman had her own small kit for grinding eye paint. The name for this important toiletry is written like the word "to protect", perhaps alluding to the ability of the make-up to keep common eye diseases at bay.[33]

Egyptian eye doctors were quite skilled, frequently implementing honey in conjunction with eye paint to treat a variety of ophthalmological disorders.[34] Research suggests that Egyptians chemically altered eye paints by mixing them with carbonated and salted waters to improve their bactericidal and protective effect. Honey would have been an ideal vehicle to deliver ground pigments, creating a relieving salve.

## SUSHRUTA: THE FATHER OF PLASTIC SURGERY

India enjoyed its own birth of medical surgery, which is often overlooked because of the difficulty of translating Sanskrit. The Vedas, the four sacred Hindu books compiled between 3,000 and 1,000 BC, contain the earliest references to Indian medical care. Hindu texts were composed in prose and orally handed down. When visiting India, Vedic chants can still be heard today. The sacred texts extol the virtues of honey: "Let one take honey … to beautify his appearance, develop his brain faculty and strengthen his body."[35]

Rational medicine took off in India with Charaka's medical treatise known as the Charaka Samhita,[36] which encompassed 120 chapters on anatomy, embryology, and dissection. Charaka is believed to have taught at the ancient university of Taksasila in north-western India around 400 BC.[37]

His contemporary Sushruta, who lived between 1,000 and 600 BC, wrote the epic text on surgery, the Sushruta Samhita, which described in detail how to reconstruct a nose and successfully complete cataract operations, along with other surgical complicated interventions. The English translation runs more than 800 pages.[38]

Together the two texts form the foundation of Ayurvedic medicine. Ayurvedic comes from the word roots *āyus*, long life, and *vedas*, knowledge. Passed down orally from one reciter to the next, both texts survived complete. In both collections, the doctors recommended a paste from a fat such as butter or ghee mixed with honey.

Sushruta practiced and taught the art of surgery. In ancient India medicinal knowledge was passed from the 'guru' (teacher) to the 'sisya' (disciple). His students trained on gourds and melons, dedicating a minimum of six years to learning the art of surgery.[39] Hindu religion taught that a dead body was sacred and could not be defiled by a knife. Sushruta figured out how to circumvent such decrees, inventing a brush-type broom that scrapped off skin and flesh without the surgeon needing to touch the corpse.[40] This enabled him to study human anatomy in detail.

Sushruta taught at the University of Benares in the ancient city of the same name in the northern part of India. The oldest living city in the world—now known as Varanasi—is considered a holy city and pilgrimage site, located on the banks of the river Ganges.

Mark Twain described the city in his book, *Following the Equator: Travels Around the World*: "Benaras is older than history, older than tradition, older even than legend and looks twice as old as all of them put together."[41] Knowledge of both surgery and medicine were essential to the success of a doctor, otherwise one "is like a bird with only one wing," wrote Sushruta.[42]

In his lyrical text, Sushruta described honey:

> *Honey is sweet, and leaves an astringent after-taste. …It acts as a purifying and healing agent in respect of ulcers and eyes, is (an)*

*aphrodisiac, astringent and tends to permeate all the minutest chan-
nels and capillaries of the organism.*[43]

The treatment of eye disorders encompasses a large section of the
Sushruta Samhita. A common procedure involved an operation for
ingrown eyelashes, a historic equivalent of an almost identical modern
day reconstructive eye surgery known as the jaeschearlt procedure:[44]

> *After being treated with sneha* (a special diet) *the patient sits
> facing the surgeon. An excision in the shape and size of barleycorn
> should be made in the eyelid horizontally parallel leaving two parts
> below the eyebrow and one part above the eyelashes. The surgeon
> should then suture up the two edges with horse's hair. An applica-
> tion of honey and ghee should be applied. A piece of linen should be
> tied around the forehead and the horse's hair sewing up the operated
> part should be attached thereto. The sutures are removed once there is
> adhesion of the two edges. If this does not succeed, cauterization of the
> upper lid or complete epilation should be performed.*[45]

The honey mixed with ghee, a clarified butter made from cow's
milk, would keep the tissue free of infection and speed the healing process. Used throughout India, ghee has all of the water and butter solids
from milk removed, and so doesn't spoil. In his medical treatise, Sushruta
proposed that the combination of ghee (*ghrita*) and honey (*madhu*) created a synergistic healing effect,[46] recommending it for the treatment of
all traumatic ulcers.[47] Ghee blends well with honey, increasing its viscosity
and stopping the honey from running out of the wound as it is diluted by
wound exudates.

Traumatic head lacerations were common occurrences and for these
Sushruta described the following treatment:

> *In a case of a fracture of the bone of the forehead unattended
> by any oozing out of brain matter, the affected part should be simply
> rubbed with honey and clarified butter and then duly bandaged.*[48]

To cure earaches, Sushruta recommended:

> *The expressed juice of green ginger, made lukewarm after mix-
> ing it with* (equal quantities of) *oil, honey and Saindhava salt, should
> be poured into the cavity of the ear in a case of* (acute) *ear-ache.*[49]

The tenth chapter of this text details how to care for pregnant and
nursing women. Sushruta recommends honey mixed with ghee as the first

food fed to a newborn. He elaborates, stating, that "the growth, memory, strength and intellect of a child are improved"[50] by the use of four medicinal potions, each of which contains honey.

To ward off evil, individuals pierced their earlobes in ancient India, enlarging the hole over time. Sushruta frequently faced torn earlobes. To reconstruct the lobe, Sushruta invented a skin graft procedure that maintained blood flow to the tissue, which was then treated with honey and ghee:

> *A surgeon well versed in the knowledge of surgery should slice off a patch of living flesh from the cheek of a person so as to have on its ends attached to its former seat* (cheek). *Then the part, where the artificial ear lobe is to be made, should be slightly scarified* (with a knife) *and the living flesh, full of blood and sliced off as previously directed, should be adhered to it* (so as to resemble a natural ear lobe in shape). *The flap should then be covered with honey and butter and bandaged with cotton and linen and dusted with the powder of baking clay.[51]*

Sushruta's most famous surgery explained how to construct a new nose, earning him fame as the world's first plastic surgeon. He invented a cheek skin transplant operation to restore amputated noses, a form a surgery in great demand. Vicious bands of marauders traipsed the countryside, inflicting facial mutilation to humiliate their victims. Most commonly they cut off the nose. This was the ultimate dishonor because one's nose was the visible embodiment of respect and reputation and its loss was mortifying.[52]

In revenge for minor offenses, the Hindu god Rama chopped off the noses of women. Hindu husbands followed the godly example, cutting off the ears and noses of their wives if they left the house without first requesting permission. Thieves, adulterers and other petty criminals sacrificed their noses when caught. Sushruta must have had a thriving business:[53]

> *When a man's nose has been cut off or destroyed, the physician takes the leaf of a plan ... He places it on the patient's cheek and cuts out of this cheek a piece of skin of the same size in such a manner that the skin at one end remains attached to the cheek... Then he freshens with his scalpel the edges of the stump of the nose and wraps the piece of skin from the cheek carefully around it and sews it at all the edges*

*...As soon as the skin has sewn together with the nose, he cuts through the connection with the cheek.*[54]

To treat infected wounds, Sushruta applied a paste of honey, clarified butter enriched with barley and four herbs.[55]

While speaking about the benefits of bee products at a state fair, a nurse mentioned to me that such ancient teachings have a modern equivalent: the plastic surgeon she works for outside of Washington, D.C. regularly uses honey to speed the healing process of his patients. The honey helps the wounds heal faster with minimal scarring.

## THE LEECHBOOK OF BALD: A PHYSICIAN'S DESK REFERENCE

One of the most detailed glimpses into Saxon herbal remedies from approximately 900 AD is the Leechbook of Bald - "leace" in Old English means healer.[56] Penned with loving care in a large, bold hand by a monk named Cild, this two volume work was a desk reference for the physician Bald, believed to be a close friend of King Alfred.[57]

In a lecture delivered by Dr. John F. Payne at the Royal College of Physicians in 1903, he described it as "the embryo of modern English medicine".[58] Unlike other texts, this compendium was composed in the vernacular instead of Latin. The author had a rich knowledge of native plants and garden herbs. Potions typically combined herbs mixed with honey. The treatise even includes a prescription for exercise for those who lacked hunger:

> *Against want of appetite. Let them, after the night's fast, lap up honey, and let them seek for themselves fatigue in riding on horseback or in a wain or such conveyance as they may endure.*[59]

The Leechbook recommends honey as a constituent of "the best eye salve", and urged use of honey for treatment of sties, dirty wounds and internal wounds, after amputations and to help the removal of scabs.[60]

The profession of leech was not easy, as patients were often purloined by the church. The clergy profited from their reputation of working miraculous cures:

> *The unfair treatment of the leech is perhaps nowhere more clearly shown than in Bede's tale of St. John of Beverly curing a boy with a diseased head. Although the leech effected the cure, the success was attributed to the bishop's benediction.*[61]

The church relished meddling in medical care, taking over the treatment of patients during the Middle Ages. The church advocated irritating substances that promoted pus formation, incorrectly believing this to be a sign of recovery.[62] Many useful treatments for wound care developed through trial and error by earlier civilizations were lost. "Wound treatment was, in effect, worse than it had been in prehistoric times."[63]

# *Interlude*

## *Democritus, the Laughing Philosopher*

Democritus, a Greek philosopher born around 450 BC in Abdera, Greece was known in antiquity as the "laughing philosopher" because he valued the personal characteristic of cheerfulness. He led a school of natural philosophers known as the Atomists, who had an astonishingly accurate view of our physical world. The belief that our macroscopic world could best be understood in terms of indivisible microscopic building blocks called atoms brought them widespread ridicule.[1]

The laughing philosopher argued against debilitating emotions like anger and hatred, cultivating instead a sense of cheerfulness and peace of mind. He lived to the ripe, old age of 109.

Athenaeus of Naucratis, the Greek gossip writer of the day, recounts the story of Democritus' death. Athenaeus gave voice to numerous famous Greeks by having them engage in dinner conversation in his 15-volume work *Deipnosophistae*, known as the *Banquet of the Learned* or *The Gastronomers*.

Written in the early part of the third century AD, he details a fictional two-day banquet in Rome where great minds and philosophers come together to debate, joke, tell anecdotes and indulge in fine foods. In 1867, James Russell Lowell wrote: "The somewhat greasy heap of a literary rag-and-bone-picker, like Athenaeus, is turned to gold by time."[2] Nevertheless, this rag-and-bone-picker, through quotes and excerpts, gives us an insight into ancient works that would otherwise have been completely lost:

> *And it is said that Democritus, the philosopher of Abdera, ...*
> *had determined to rid himself of old age. ...He had begun to dimin-*

*ish his food day by day, when the day of the Thesmophorian festival came round, and the women of his household besought him not to die during the festival, in order that they might not be debarred from their share in the festivities; (he) was persuaded, and ordered a vessel full of honey to be set near him: and in this way he lived many days with no other support than honey; and then some days after, when the honey had been taken away, he died. But Democritus had always been fond of honey; and he once answered a man, who asked him how he could live in the enjoyment of the best health, that he might do so if he constantly moistened his inward parts with honey and his outward man with oil.*

Perhaps Democritus was on to something, for the word "*medicine*" derives from the word-root *medu* - used in most Indo-European languages to describe honey or drinks made from honey:

*mead* in English,
*medd* in Welsh,
*mede* in Dutch,
*mjød* in Danish,
*mjod* in Russian, and
*madhu* in Sanskrit.

The word root "medu" suggests honey has been tied to healing since antiquity. It seems fitting therefore that Democritus—the honey-loving philosopher—was buried in honey.[3]

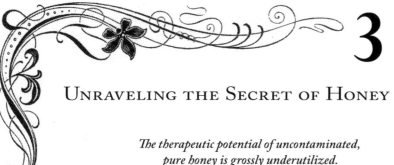

# 3

## Unraveling the Secret of Honey

*The therapeutic potential of uncontaminated,
pure honey is grossly underutilized.
...The time has now come for conventional medicine
to lift the blinds off this 'traditional remedy'
and give it its due recognition.*

- Zumla and Lulat, 1989,
Journal of the Royal Society of Medicine

*O*ur ancestors enjoyed the medicinal benefits of honey long before we had a written language. Doctors liberally applied honey to a variety of ailments, curing infections and speeding up the healing process. With the advent of antibiotics in the early 1940s honey disappeared from conventional western medicine. Now that antibiotics fail against resistant superbugs on a regular basis, honey has surged back into the limelight as a cost-effective, efficient and surprisingly successful remedy.

Hippocrates, Aristotle, and Pliny, amongst numerous other great minds and medical practitioners, recognized the therapeutic potential of honey. They all applied it liberally to open wounds. "It causes heat, cleans sores and ulcers, softens hard ulcers of the lip, heals carbuncles and running sores," wrote Hippocrates.[1]

In ancient papyri, as we have seen, medical doctors recorded hundreds of prescriptions containing the ingredient honey for external and internal applications. Frequently the authors listed a host of substitutes for individual ingredients, indicating a wide variety of materials would suffice. But they were adamant in their need for honey, rarely suggesting an alternative.[2] Our ancestors knew honey worked; nothing else would do.

## THE STERILE HIVE

A honey bee hive is a warm, moist environment with up to 60,000 inhabitants living in an extremely compact space - the ideal atmosphere for bacteria to flourish. But surprisingly enough, they don't. The products of the hive—honey, propolis, royal jelly, bee bread and beeswax—each have properties to inhibit the growth of harmful microbes.

## HONEY: NATURE'S ANTIMICROBIAL SOLUTION

As a super-saturated sugar solution, honey is an ideal antimicrobial agent. In the first part of last century, a bacteriologist by the name of Walter G. Sackett decided to investigate honey bees while working at the Colorado State University Agricultural Experimental Station. Like his father before him, who had once condemned the water supply of Fort Collins, CO to the chagrin of city officials, Dr. Sackett studied how diseases could be spread.

After seeing bees buzzing around an outdoor privy, Dr. Sackett wanted to learn if these prolific pollinators could spread maladies such as typhoid fever and dysentery. To his surprise, he discovered that bacteria added to honey were killed. Strangely enough, when the honey was diluted with water, it was even more effective at eliminating bacteria. In 1919 he was the first American to report honey's antibacterial properties.[3] Apparently the Dutch scientist Van Ketel had beaten him to the finish line, reporting on honey's bactericidal properties back in 1892.[4]

While doctors of antiquity clearly valued the benefits of honey, they did not understand how it worked. This seemingly simple question remained unsolved for thousands of years until 1937, when a curiously named trio called Dold, Du and Dziao unraveled part of the mystery.[5] Working in a research lab in Germany, they discovered honey killed certain common bacteria, especially when diluted with water. Stumped and unable to uncover the identity of this antibacterial substance, they dubbed the enigma "inhibine"; a tribute to its inhibitory effects on microbial growth.

## SIR ALEXANDER FLEMING AND THE QUEST FOR PENICILLIN

Less than a decade beforehand in 1928, a Scottish scientist toiled away in his laboratory buried in the basement of St. Mary's Hospital in London. Although quite brilliant, he often forgot about his culture plates; little petri dishes growing colonies of bacteria. When he returned from a long vacation he discovered his plates contaminated by blue-green mold. Thinking they were useless, he prepared to clean them out but a visitor asked to see his work so the genial Sir Alexander Fleming retrieved one of his moldy plates. When he did he noticed a clear circle surrounding the fuzzy mold. Where the mold touched the bacteria it stopped the microbes in their tracks. Sir Fleming had discovered penicillin.

Penicillin proved to be a finicky substance that was very difficult to isolate and produce en masse. After a few unsuccessful attempts to isolate the antibiotic substance, Fleming gave up the quest.

From Fleming's discovery in 1928, it would take over a decade to mass produce penicillin. To turn penicillin into a functioning medicine took a dedicated group of researchers at Oxford, led by the driven Dr. Florey, and monumental support from giant pharmaceutical companies in the United States. Only through this massive cooperation could penicillin be developed, thus launching the antibiotic craze.

Huge laboratories produced large quantities of penicillin from vast batches of mold broth in the early 1940s, making it cheap and widely available. Doctors prescribed it with gusto. In 1947, after four short years of undefeated stardom, the superhero penicillin lost its first battle against the common bacteria *Staphylococcus aureus*, frequently called staph.

But by that time researchers had developed a new antibiotic to replace penicillin and the antibiotic race was on. Scientists clamored to create ever better antibiotics. Struggling to survive against the onslaught of poisons, bacteria quickly developed resistance to each new antibiotic substance.

In 1969, the U.S. Surgeon General William H. Stewart thought antibiotics had won the battle and confidently informed Congress we can "close the book on infectious disease".[6] Much like the head of the patent office, who allegedly claimed in 1899 that his department should be shut down because "everything that can be invented has been invented", he was utterly wrong!

## Unraveling the Mysterious Inhibines

With antibiotics in vogue, interest in and funding for research looking into more complex natural substances like honey all but dried up. In 1942, while Hitler steamrolled over his neighbors, Jonathan W. White, Jr.,[7] a thin man with a strong hawkish nose and dark rimmed glasses finished framing his doctoral degree from Purdue University in agricultural chemistry. Although he had worked for the USDA since 1942, he put his career on hold in 1944, moving to Washington, D.C. to help in the war effort as an employee in the U.S. Bureau of Censorship.[8] After the end of the war, the young scientist returned to his post at the USDA Eastern Regional Research Laboratory in Wyndmoor, Pennsylvania, where he dedicated his life to understanding the complexity of the world's original sweetener.

Eighteen long years passed before USDA honey scientist extraordinaire Dr. White untangled the mystery of those secretive inhibines in honey. While working as Head of Honey Investigations, White discovered honey acquires much of its antibacterial punch from an enzyme bees add called glucose oxidase. This enzyme sits quite demurely in honey, much like an obedient child raised before the tumultuous 1960s who was to be seen but not heard. But add a little water and this enzyme springs into action, reacting with the water molecules to form gluconic acid and minute amounts of hydrogen peroxide.

As many know, hydrogen peroxide was once welcomed by the medical community with great applause as a fantastic healer, but then faded from the stage as it damaged tissue. In contrast, the continuous production of weak hydrogen peroxide from honey—at approximately 1/1000 of the strength of the store bought three percent solution[9]—helps heal without any negative drawbacks.

## Breeding Superbugs

Unlike honey, antibiotics have a single mechanism for eliminating microbes: they attack the bacteria's cell wall or inhibit the internal functioning of the cell by scrambling important intracellular metabolic pathways, in effect poisoning the pathogens. Some bacterial mutations immune to the poison survive. These resistant microbes reproduce, passing on their resistance and creating strains of almost impossible to eliminate superbugs that wreak havoc in hospitals and homes. "Lurking in our homes, hospitals, schools and farms is a terrifying pathogen that is evolving faster than the medical community can track it or drug developers can create antibiotics to quell it. That pathogen is MRSA—methicillin-resistant *Staphylococcus aureus*,"[10] a deadly superbug.

Unintentionally we are selectively breeding virulent bacteria by constantly exposing them to antibiotics. Our overuse of antibiotics "culls out" bacteria with little resistance, so only the fittest, most resistant strains survive.

The genes that give bacteria resistance are ancient genes that evolved in the distant past when bacteria and fungi were competing for resources. In a battle of survival, they tried to kill each other, trying to outsmart their would-be assassins before they were eliminated themselves. Darwin's survival of the fittest also plays out on these miniscule living organisms. Those better suited for survival produce more offspring, passing their small survival advantages on to the next generation, which add up over time.

## SWEET AND SOUR

Always thirsty, the sugars of honey pull water out of the surrounding environment in a process scientists call osmotic action. This hygroscopic action sucks the water and life out of bacteria. So any mutations that give the bacteria increased resistance to antibiotics are eliminated.

The acidic pH of honey, which sways from 3.2-4.5 depending on the type of honey,[11] also stops bacteria from thriving.

The sugar content alone is not the sole reason for honey's antibacterial properties. When researchers mix up an artificial honey that mimics the natural sugar content of honey, it performs poorly in comparison to the real product in the battle against microbes. Minute concentrations of active honey will stop a wide range of bacteria, but you need five to ten times as much artificial honey. Clearly more is at work than simple sugars.

## THE DELICATE TOUCH OF HYDROGEN PEROXIDE

Honey's potency swells when diluted; the increased water content frees glucose oxidase to react and create hydrogen peroxide. This reduces the sugar content, eliminating the osmotic action. Yet the watered down honey still eliminates common staph bacteria with its unremitting release of hydrogen peroxide. Taken together, honey's natural antibacterial properties inhibit the growth of approximately 60 species of bacteria, including aerobes and anaerobes, gram-positives and gram-negatives.[12]

A natural product, honey varies widely in its antibacterial potency. Some samples can have a hundred times more potency than others.[13,14] Exposure to light or heat destroys the enzyme glucose oxidase, responsible for the production of the helpful hydrogen peroxide. Consumers in the United States prefer clear, liquid honey. To satisfy this desire, honey processors heat honey to high temperatures, so that it won't crystallize quickly - a death sentence for heat sensitive glucose oxidase.

If you desire antibacterial activity in your honey, it is best to use raw (unpasteurized) honey. There is no need to pasteurize honey, as the bacteria that are killed by pasteurization can't survive the high sugar content of honey. Pasteurization will only kill the harmless yeasts, which would allow honey to ferment under certain conditions.

## POWER OF THE PLANTS

While we imagine leaf munching animals to be the greatest predator of plants, microbes and fungi boast a much more voracious appetite for green growing vegetation. In the plant world, Darwin's survival of the fittest plays out at a microscopic level. To fend off starving microorganisms, plants develop protective chemicals which course through the equivalent of their bodies. Some of these shielding properties exist in the nectar bees turn into honey.

Honey made from the nectar of a variety of tea tree shrub found in New Zealand and Australia wields a potent antibacterial weapon. Bees visit the profusely blooming manuka and jellybush shrubs, gathering nectar from the delicate bright white or soft pink flowers that sink into deep blood purple centers. Dr. Peter Molan from the University of Waikato in New Zealand discovered that honey made from manuka trees contains a light and heat stable component that eliminates microbes even when researchers have disabled the hydrogen peroxide content in honey.

To test a honey for additional antibacterial properties, researchers simply add a different enzyme called catalase, which destroys the hydrogen peroxide. After knocking out the hydrogen peroxide activity, manuka and jellybush honey still inhibit bacteria.

The human body can also produce catalase, which could eliminate much of the hydrogen peroxide production of honey. The high sugar content and acidity of honey still help stop bacterial growth in the presence of catalase, but this action decreases as fluids from the wound dilute the honey; so antibacterial properties immune to catalase are vital in wound healing as the body can not degrade them.

## The Magic of Manuka

Manuka honey has garnered much attention in the last decade for its superb wound healing abilities. But this honey used to languish in obscurity and beekeepers had trouble selling harvests of manuka honey because consumers found the honey's strong, astringent taste unpalatable. Only native New Zealanders, the Maori, carried knowledge of manuka honey's antiseptic properties in their folklore.

The veil of obscurity was ripped off manuka honey in 1982, when Dr. Peter Molan at the University of Waikato in New Zealand discovered manuka honey had a unique, heat-stable antibacterial activity making it ideal for wound healing. This same quality was later uncovered in Australian jellybush honey by Dr. Craig Davis in the Department of Primary Industries in Queensland, Australia. Unlike other honeys, this activity is not caused by the production of hydrogen peroxide from the enzyme glucose oxidase.

Dr. Molan's discovery and his subsequent years of research on manuka's wound healing properties fuelled interest in this honey. As demand for manuka honey grew around the world, it revitalized the New Zealand beekeeping industry and sales continue to escalate.

For years researchers tried to uncover the elusive ingredient that bestowed manuka and jellybush honeys powerful antibacterial clout. Over a hundred elements were candidates for the potent antibacterial properties.

In the summer of 2007, a German scientist from the University of Dresden declared methylgloxal (MGO) the magic ingredient. Had the decade old mystery finally been solved?

A trio from the world's foremost honey research lab at the University of Waikato completed 25 years of research and confirmed methylgloxal did indeed endow manuka honey with its potency in early 2008. Another mystery in the long history of honey had been solved - or so it seemed.

However, MGO levels are misleading, as they do not have a direct correlation to the antibacterial potency of the honey. "Something in manuka honey, without any antibacterial activity of its own, acts as a synergist with the MGO to create an effect greater than that predicted by knowing only the separate effect of the MGO,"[15] Dr. Peter Molan explained.

At low levels, MGO acts in synergy with other components of the honey, producing relatively high levels of antibacterial activity. However, the synergy only works to a certain point. To attain even higher rates of antibacterial potency you need dramatically higher levels of MGO, which makes it a deceptive reference point for judging the activity level of a honey. A honey with twice the MGO level does not have twice the antibacterial activity, so selling active manuka honey by the MGO content misleads consumers.

## TESTED RATING SYSTEM

After working with manuka honey for several years, Dr. Molan developed a Unique Manuka Factor (UMF) rating system to judge the level of antibacterial activity in each batch of manuka honey. To be considered an "active" honey, the batch should have a rating of 10 or more. The number matches the antibacterial potency of the standard antiseptic phenol, also known as carbolic. So a UMF honey with a rating of 10 has the same activity as a 10 percent solution of the standard antiseptic. For medicinal purposes such as the treatment of infected wounds in hospitals, doctors should apply a honey with a UMF rating from 12 to 16.

The UMF system is trademarked and only members of the Active Manuka Honey Association (AMHA) may use it. Over the years AMHA has become a rather exclusive organization. Non-members may not use the registered trademark, leaving many manuka honey packers and producers without an identifiable standard to label their product. A profusion of labels touting different forms of activity have entered the marketplace, confusing consumers.

To help stem the flood of rating systems and alleviate the bewilderment, Dr. Molan created the Molan Gold Standard rating system. As with the UMF system, the number on the honey label corresponds to the activity of a similar phenol solution.

## BON VOYAGE BACTERIA

Numerous different types of bacteria can not survive in the presence of honey. Yet many of these same pathogens cause serious ailments, including stomach ulcers, pneumonia and cholera. In lab tests honey has stopped cold all of these potentially harmful bacteria:

## Pathogens Honey Eliminates

| Pathogen | Infection it causes |
|---|---|
| *Bacillus anthracis* | Anthrax |
| *Corynebacterium diphtheria* | Diptheria |
| *Haemophilus influenza* | Ear infections, meningitis, respiratory infections, sinusitis |
| *Helicobacter pylori* | Ulcers, stomach cancer, sudden death syndrome |
| *Klebsiella pneumonia* | Pneumonia |
| *Listeria monocytogenes* | Meningitis |
| *Mycobacterium tuberculosis* | Tuberculosis |
| *Pasteurella multocida* | Infected animal bites |
| *Proteus species* | Septicemia, urinary infections, wound infections |
| *Pseudomonas aeruginosa* | Urinary infections, wound infections |
| *Salmonella species* | Diarrhea |
| *Salmonella cholera-suis* | Septicemia |
| *Salmonella typhi* | Typhoid fever |
| *Salmonella typhimurium* | Wound infections, gastroenteritis |
| *Serratia marcescens* | Septicemia, wound infections |
| *Shigella species* | Dysentery |
| *Staphylococcus aureus* | Abscesses, boils, carbuncles, impetigo, wound infections |
| *Streptococcus faecalis* | Urinary infections |
| *Streptococcus mutans* | Dental caries |
| *Streptococcus pneumoniae* | Ear infections, meningitis, pneumonia, sinusitis |
| *Streptococcus pyogenes* | Ear infections, impetigo, puerperal fever, rheumatic fever, scarlet fever, sore throat, wound infections |
| *Vibrio cholera* | Cholera |

This table is taken from an article published by honey expert and researcher Dr. Peter Molan.[16]

## HONEY—THE GROSSLY UNDERUTILIZED ANTIMICROBIAL

With a cheerful smile, the vibrant redhead Dr. Shona Blair, a microbiologist who studies the effect of honey on pathogens, started her talk at the first International Symposium on Honey and Human Health in 2008 by noting honey's long history. "Any culture that had access to honey used it for medicinal purposes," she said, as her favorite cave painting appeared on the screen behind her. "This painting dates from 8,000 BC and it is the first example of humans using fire to harvest honey. The size of the hive, seen from the bottom, dominates the man, attributing greater significance to the honey."

Throughout the ages we used honey extensively for trauma and surgical wounds. "The advent of antibiotics in the early 1940s killed the use of honey. Antibiotics are marvelous drugs. They have saved millions of lives, but unfortunately we overuse them." This overuse permits the development of resistance and the World Health Organization has stated we need to minimize our antibiotic use.

"Once we cut back on antibiotics by using alternatives such as honey, the resistant pathogens disappear and the antibiotics regain their effects," Dr. Blair explained, her eyes sparkling with enthusiasm.

Most antibacterial products delay healing, but quite the reverse happens with antibacterial honey. This ancient remedy helps eliminate inflammation and supports the formation of new tissue.

Some doctors argue the antimicrobial effects of honey are due solely to its high sugar content, which pulls moisture out of bacteria. Dr. Blair displayed row after row of pathogens next to the percentages required to inhibit their growth. While active manuka honey, or a honey rich in glucose oxidase, eliminated a long list of microbial growth at four percent concentrations, an artificial honey with identical sugar composition to normal honey needed a 20-25 percent concentration to achieve the same effects.

In Dr. Blair's experience honey proved effective against 1) chronic acne, a debilitating disease linked to depression and increased suicide; 2) thrush, a painful oral yeast infection; 3) wounds, especially those infected by resistant bacteria; 4) biofilms, communities of microbes that form a protective layer of slime and love setting up shop on indwelling medical devices such as catheters or pins inserted in limbs.

"Biofilms can pack 1,000 times more resistance than the same strain of microorganism living free," Dr. Blair said. "Chronic wounds and diabetic ulcers often have resident biofilms that keep them from healing."

She has discovered that these biofilms are extremely susceptible to honey. Even minute amounts of honey (one percent concentration) caused a drop in biofilm activity. A five percent honey solution completely eliminated these otherwise resilient colonies.

"My loved ones know that if I'm in an accident and I die, they should donate my organs. If I live, they should cover me with honey."

## ANTIFUNGAL POTENTIAL

Some honeys inhibit fungal growth. Honey has great potential for eliminating yeast infections, which are often caused by Candida species. The most common invader answers to the name of *Candida albicans*. When it gets out of hand it can cause vaginal yeast infections, thrush, diaper rash and nail bed infections.

The dermatophytes are another group of fungi that create problems when they set up home on our bodies, causing jock itch, ringworm and athlete's foot. As anyone who has had a bout with these types of superficial fungal infections knows, they can be a pain to eliminate. Antibiotics are practically ineffective against fungal colonies. Research shows active honeys have the potential to eliminate pesky fungal infections at five to 25 percent concentrations.[17]

During conversation, Dr. Shona Blair divulged her potent healing cream recipe, where she mixes two parts unscented cream to one part active honey - a similar ratio used by ancient healers. This soothing cream eliminates the stickiness of honey, making it easy to apply. The mixture ensures a honey dilution of 33 percent, more than enough to eradicate difficult fungal infections. She recounted how it proved effective for a colleague who had suffered from jock itch since he attended boarding school at the age of 15. She has also used it successfully against athlete's foot and sunburn.

Clinical trials confirming the potential of antifungal salves are needed, but the first results look promising. Honey creams may soon become stock items in sweaty, wet locker rooms, where fungal infections love to spread.

## Honey's Multifaceted Benefits

- **Osmotic action:** high sugar content of honey dehydrates bacteria

- **High acidity:** stops microbial growth of pathogenic bacteria

- **Glucose oxidase:** slow, continuous release of hydrogen peroxide acts as potent antibiotic; also stimulates wound debridement

- **Non-peroxide activity:** heat stable antibacterial activity

- **Moist wound environment**: helps tissues heal faster

- **Anti-inflammatory properties**: soothes and relieves inflammation

- **Antioxidants:** promote good health and longevity

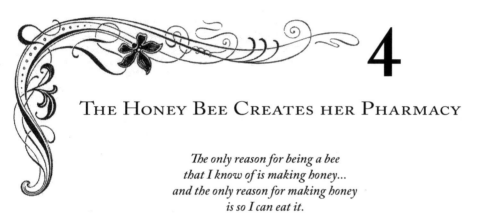

# 4

## THE HONEY BEE CREATES HER PHARMACY

*The only reason for being a bee
that I know of is making honey...
and the only reason for making honey
is so I can eat it.*

- Winnie the Pooh

*F*or us to enjoy a single pound of honey, worker bees must fly over 55,000 miles, collecting nectar from approximately two million blossoms. The bees that do all the work in the hive are females. Instead of investing energy in raising their own young, these worker bees forage for food and raise the young of their mother, the queen.

Bees have existed for over a hundred million years. In their long shared history, insect pollinators and flowers evolved in a symbiotic arms race. The flowers developed ever more elaborate schemes to lure pollinators with vibrant color palettes and sweet offerings of nectar, while the insects evolved to exploit the resources on offer. Bees helped usher in the rapid diversification and dominance of these flowering plants, known as angiosperms.[1] In 2006 scientists analyzed the oldest known bee fossil entombed in one-hundred-million-year-old amber, discovering the bee collected pollen - an ancient relative of the modern honey bee.

In the battle to win the sweet caresses of a pollinator, flowers also developed unique markings to guide fly-by pollinators to the sugary reward. As the bees dart through the air, they scan the ground below with their compound eyes, but they do not see the same world we do. Lit by the ultra-violet light of the sun, their view from above looks quite different from ours.

While we admire the beauty of a bold red poppy or an airy white daisy, the honey bee sees the flower's ultra-violet markings. These ultra-violet streaks engrave the colorful petals like road markings on airport runways, directing pollinators toward hidden bounties of nectar.[2] Once nectar seekers deplete the sugary resource, the ultra-violet nectar guides of some plants fade away, informing the passing pollinator to look elsewhere.

Honey bees, *Apis mellifera* or *mellifica* the "honey carrier" or "honey maker", do so much more than simply make honey. These industrious creatures are prolific pollinators. Instead of being choosy and restricting its foraging to a few specific plants, the honey bee is a generalist, visiting a wide variety of blooms in search of sweet carbohydrates (nectar) and protein (pollen). Both the plant and the insect benefit from this interaction, a relationship known as mutualism. (For an interesting review of how this relationship has become endangered see Kearns, Inouye et al. 1998).

Flying through the air, honey bees pick up an electrostatic charge. When they land on a flower, pollen grains from the flower's male anther literally jump onto the bees' hairy body. Honey bees, in effect, suffer from constant static cling.

Like all good females, honey bee foragers have figured out how to deal with this problem. The little ladies always travel with a comb to deal with bad hair days. Covered in pollen, they moisten their legs with nectar or water and run them along their body, gathering the loose pollen grains. Using the comb built into their third and final pair of legs, they brush the collected pollen into a big sticky ball. They then press the mass into a neat little package about the size of a single piece of Grape Nut cereal using a notch on this hind leg. Masters of efficiency, they store this colorful little ball in their nifty pollen baskets called corbicula.

Bees travel from flower to flower, gathering nectar and pollen. At each landing a few pollen grains fall off, often as they scurry into the depths of the flower to sup nectar. Male pollen grains drop onto the female stigma, connected to the plant's ovary - successful plant sex through a third party. The industrious honey bee provides pollination to numerous plants and agricultural crops. Her labors result in increased agricultural product quality and quantity valued at $14 billion annually in the United States.

Pollination is big business. Beekeepers load up 1.5 million hives every year from as far away as Florida and truck them cross country to the verdant almond orchards of California to cash in on pollination fees. Pollination is so important, even Albert Einstein is supposed to have weighed in with this perceptive statement:

> *If the bee disappeared off the surface of the globe, then man would only have four years of life left: no bees, no pollination, no plants, no animals, no people...*

Every third bite of food that crosses our lips is either directly or indirectly pollinated by the honey bee, which makes this little, maligned insect a marvel. Without honey bees, we would not produce our beloved cranberries, almonds, oranges, concurbits, apples, pears, cherries, blueberries, and a host of other fruits and vegetables in the quantity and quality we currently enjoy. All together bees pollinate over 90 different agricultural crops.

Some may scoff at the loss of fruits and vegetables, but without the honey bee, we jeopardize our dairy supplies. The lactating animals need a rich diet of clover and alfalfa. Only through honey bees can we produce enough clover and alfalfa seed to plant our lush hay fields. The U.S. value of pollination attributed to honey bees far surpasses the current value of all bee hive products produced. Let's take a closer look at how bees make honey.

## NECTAR: THE RAW MATERIAL FOR HONEY

To produce the sugary reward of nectar, plants must first make glucose. By harvesting the energy of the sun using photosynthesis, plants convert carbon dioxide and water into glucose and oxygen. The conversion occurs in chlorophyll, a protein found abundantly in plant chloroplasts which congregate in plant leaves. Some of the glucose is then converted into sap and transported via the sieve tubes of the phloem tissue to storage organs. A portion of the sap ends up as nectar in the flower, enticing bees to visit.

Nectar is a rich carbohydrate composed of the two simple sugars fructose and glucose along with the more complex sugar sucrose. The type of plant determines the ratio of the three sugars and influences the sugar concentration. An area's climate also sways the sugar concentration. Not surprisingly the hot, dry environments of deserts often produce more concentrated nectar, while moist, cool climates can lower the sugar concentration and increase the water content. But despite the climate, a few species of plants will produce concentrated nectars in damp conditions and thin, watery nectars in dry climates. In addition to sugars and water, nectar also contains aromatic esters, minerals, vitamins and amino acids; all of which sculpt the taste of a given honey.

## HONEYDEW

Bees are not picky. They will collect just about any sweet material they can carry home. I know of a beekeeper who keeps an apiary near a Domino Sugar factory. In years past the hives have produced a honey with the distinct aroma of molasses. A beekeeper in Germany once extracted a honey in a shade of lime green. His bees had stumbled upon an open source of verdant Waldmeister - sweet, bright green woodruff syrup, making a honey in the shade of new leaves.

Besides the sweet man-made anomalies bees sometimes encounter, foragers will collect honeydew. Honeydew is the sugary secretion of insects that gorge on the phloem sap of plants. Only a select group of insects engage in this behavior, including aphids, scale insects and some members of the suborder *Auchenorrhycha*. Using their mouthparts, these insects pierce into plant tissue until they penetrate the phloem arteries. The internal pressure then forces the sap out of the punctured plant tissue, so that the insect need only drink. The phloem sap contains sugars, peptides and many other important elements that nourish the feeding insect.

In most insects the imbibed sap enters the digestive tract, where enzymes are added and the sap is altered by the microflora inhabiting the insect's gut. These beneficial microflora feed on small portions of the sap, generating important amino acids and vitamins that help sustain the insect. The concentrated sugary fluid is then excreted in a crystal clear drop. Ants and bees harvest this sugary substance. Some insects like aphids produce honeydew to garner the protection of ants, which in return deter the aphids' predator - the ladybug.

## Transforming Nectar or Honeydew into Honey

Come early spring, blossoms open their petals, offering up carbohydrate rich nectar to passing pollinators. Forager honey bees dart out of the safety of their hive to gather this sugary substance. *Apis mellifera* have evolved a series of specialized tools to carry home the bounty from blossoms.

On each of its hind legs, the worker bee has a concave region with specialized hairs that form a pollen basket, known as a corbicula, for transporting a packed pellet of pollen back to the hive. Bees also have a nectar crop, a large carrying tank located below the esophagus and above the digestive tract for hauling home the sugary reward. The nectar crop has a one-way valve,[3,4,5] which prevents nectar that has entered the midgut from returning to the nectar crop,[6] earning it the name "honey-stopper".[7] If the bee needs energy during her foraging trip, she can pass some nectar through the valve into the ventriculus (midgut), where it is digested and absorbed.

A worker bee can carry approximately 25-40 mg of nectar back to the hive; a load about the size of a large raindrop. To gather a full load of nectar a forager visits one to 500 flowers on a single trip. Instead of skipping from one type of flower to another, the bee sups from only one type of flower, never switching varieties during her trip. Such loyal behavior has its own term - floral fidelity and serves the plant very well; it wouldn't benefit an apple blossom to have its male pollen transported to the female parts of a pear blossom.

Floral fidelity also benefits the beekeeper and the gourmet honey connoisseur. To harvest honey, beekeepers need a *nectar flow*, a term used to describe an abundance of nectar producing flowers in bloom. Only when a large nectar source is available will bees produce enough extra honey for the beekeeper to take a share. By giving the bees extra storage boxes on top of the brood nest at just the right time, beekeepers encourage their ladies to gather more nectar.

If the bee stumbles across an abundant nectar source, the successful forager recruits others to the find upon her return home. She reenters the hive and unloads her harvest to her hive sisters. If this happens quickly, the bee realizes she carried home a prized harvest and dances enthusiastically. An abstract language, the dance communicates to her hive mates the direction and distance of the nectar bounty. They fly out following her directions and carry home more nectar, dancing enthusiastically to recruit even more foragers to the source. Dr. Karl von Frisch decoded this unusual form of communication, garnering the Nobel Prize for his efforts.

Should the nectar flow last long enough, the bees will produce a honey from that predominant nectar source and the beekeeper will harvest a varietal honey with a distinctive taste, such as sourwood, basswood or alfalfa. The bee imbibes the nectar or honeydew drop with her proboscis. If the nectar is too thick, she may first thin it with secretions from special glands in her mouth and head. As the nectar travels down her esophagus into the honey crop, the bee mixes in additional secretions from glands, which help convert the nectar into honey.

Honey, sometimes described as summer's sunshine, is not equivalent to dehydrated nectar. As a bee struggles back to the hive, she adds enzymes to her load. Back at the hive, the successful forager waits for a hive mate to unload her nectar. She will offer a taste to receiving workers. If her cargo is deemed to meet current colony needs, and food storers are available to relieve her, she will quickly discharge her load. When her crop contents are less desirable, the honey storage areas are full, or the food storer bees are engaged, it will take a long time for her to successfully deliver her nectar crop.[8,9] Instead of passing the whole content to a single worker, she will usually share the bounty among many.

Once the nectar is passed to the first receiver bee, it has begun its long journey within the hive to become honey. The receiver bee passes the nectar to another hive bee, a process repeated numerous times. Each worker adds enzymes like invertase - a protein that breaks sucrose down into the simple sugars fructose and glucose, diastase, glucose oxidase and phosphatase, as well as the amino acid proline.[10] The addition of enzymes physically changes the properties of the nectar, helping to turn it into honey.

As the nectar is passed from bee to bee, more enzymes are added and excess moisture is evaporated off. Slower nectar flows are processed more completely than massive nectar flows. During a massive nectar flow, the bees stash their loads quickly and move onto the next. Hasty storage of the nectar in the honeycomb cells means it receives less thorough processing. The more bees involved—the longer the chain from the nectar's arrival at the hive entrance until its storage in the final honey cell—the better the manipulation that converts nectar into honey.

In each bee, microbial commensals that inhabit the honey stomach interact with the nectar. Twelve different types of lactic acid bacteria have been identified in the honey bee stomach.[11] These beneficial lactic acid bacteria (LAB) produce antimicrobial acids, hydrogen peroxide and antimicrobial peptides that protect their hosts from harmful microorganisms.[12]

Hive bees actively dry down the nectar, fanning out a nectar drop repeatedly in their mouthparts, like a woman opening and closing a pocket fan. This behavior creates a greater surface area that dries out faster.[13] The bees transfer the nectar from one cell to another. This continual movement causes much of the moisture content to evaporate in steam. Nectar that may have had as much as 80 percent water will be dried down to 20-30 percent moisture.

Finally the bees pack the almost ripe honey into cells, but it is still not honey. Masters of architecture, the bees build hexagonal cells in the hive using the least amount of material to store the most amount of honey. Built on an incline of approximately nine degrees, the cells slope upward so the moist nectar does not run out.

The cell remains uncapped for some time yet. To complete the ripening, the bees form long drooping chains, a living thread of bees, one clasped onto another. By chaining and then fanning their wings, the hive bees set up airstreams that circulate warm air throughout the hive, evaporating moisture.

When raising young in the spring through fall, the bees maintain a temperature of 97° F in their nursery, which beekeepers call the brood nest. The heat from this toasty warm environment rises, ensuring that the nectar stored in the combs above continues to passively lose moisture. When a worker bee determines that the honey has achieved the desired viscosity, she closes off the cell with a beeswax capping. Usually this occurs when the honey has reached less than 18 percent moisture.

The transformation of nectar or honeydew into honey thus requires the following steps:

- addition of enzymes: invertase, diastase, glucose oxidase and phosphatases

- addition of other substances that originate in the bee's internal glands

- lowering the pH through the production of acids in the honey stomach

- evaporation of water

- changes to the chemical composition, especially the sugar

ratios as invertase splits the disaccharide sucrose into the two simple sugars glucose and fructose

Honey provides the bees with a ready source of carbohydrates during times of dearth. Because of its high sugar content, low pH and enzyme content, honey does not spoil. It inhibits the growth of microorganisms that would be harmful to the stores or colony and thus serves as an ideal larder filled during times of plenty.

## Varietal Honeys

Most beekeepers harvest a wildflower honey, which the bees gather from a medley of blooming trees, shrubs and flowers. However, some beekeepers make the extra effort to harvest varietal honeys, which means they take advantage of the bee's floral fidelity and extract honey produced predominantly from one variety of plant.

A true gourmand understands that honey comes in an amazing parade of shades and flavors, almost equaling the diversity of wine. Just like wine, the tones of a particular honey will be different from year to year, depending on hive locations, nectar abundance and prevailing weather conditions.

Perhaps at some point in time, when more connoisseurs become aware of the uniqueness of this sweet delicacy, a first-class vintage of honey will be stored in a honey cellar for future enjoyment and a premium price. In the meantime, try tantalizing your palate by enjoying the delicate tones of black locust, the minty flavor of eucalyptus, or the robust, forest notes of red birch honeydew.

Honeys made from diverse floral sources not only have distinctive tastes, they also have varying medicinal properties. Every country has an abundance of folklore recommending particular honey types for specific ailments. The healers from the past may well have been right. New research shows that certain honeys have different beneficial properties; some are higher in antibacterial activity, others have more antioxidants, some more vigorously promote tissue repair. Only additional research will elucidate the full spectrum of the bee's bounty.

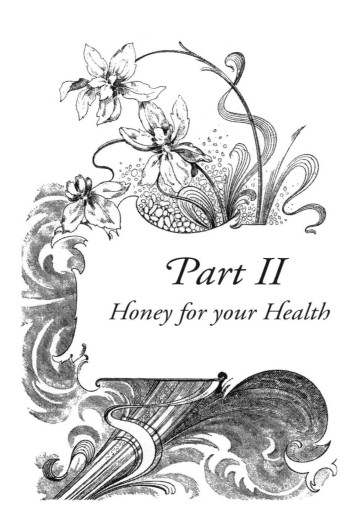

# Part II
## *Honey for your Health*

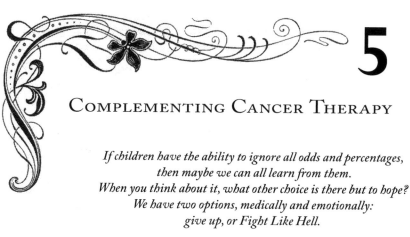

# COMPLEMENTING CANCER THERAPY

*If children have the ability to ignore all odds and percentages,*
*then maybe we can all learn from them.*
*When you think about it, what other choice is there but to hope?*
*We have two options, medically and emotionally:*
*give up, or Fight Like Hell.*

- Lance Armstrong

*We* all wish for miracles. Sweet honey with its ability to eliminate superbugs, heal chronic wounds and reduce inflammation surpasses many prescription drugs, but everything has its limits. With its potent free radical scavenging ability, honey may help prevent cancer, but once established, nature's first sweetener has not been shown to cure cancer. However, for those battling the deadly disease, it may be able to help you—in the words of Lance Armstrong—"fight like hell" against the odds. Honey has certainly improved the quality of life for cancer patients.

In the United States half of all men will develop some form of cancer in their lifetime. Women face slightly better odds of one in three.[1] We all have friends or family, who fight hard against this debilitating disease. In 2011, cancer will kill 571,950 Americans.[2] That's over 1,500 people each and every day; the second leading cause of death in America. Only heart disease claims more lives.

While we often refer to cancer as a disease of civilization, it has occurred throughout the ages. The first description of tumor like growths in breasts exists in the Edwin Smith Papyrus dedicated to the treatment of battle wounds. Breast cancer today occurs much more frequently in women, but this ancient Egyptian document details the ailment in a man[3] and concludes there is nothing the surgeon can do; it is *a medical condition you will not be able to treat.*[4] Cancer has probably existed almost as long as the human race, but the number afflicted with the disease has soared in the last century.

In our bodies, healthy cells divide, creating new ones to replace worn out and dying cells. Cell replication occurs rapidly in our youth and slows down as we mature. As adults the cells divide at a normal pace, replacing dead cells. Cell division also springs into action to repair injuries, replacing impaired cells with new, fully functioning ones.

Free radicals damage DNA, which regulates cell behavior and replication. Usually an impaired cell can no longer reproduce, so when it dies, the broken DNA also ceases to exist. But sometimes the DNA mutation does not affect the replication instructions, so the cell can still reproduce itself. Now instead of creating an identical copy of a healthy cell, it creates malfunctioning cells. These faulty cells then create duplicates of themselves. Cancer cells often have mutations that remove the multiple brake systems that stop a cell from entering the replication cycle. Essentially broken, the cancer cells just keep dividing and replicating. These rapidly reproducing cells clump together, forming a tumor.

Some tumors are benign, causing little damage because they stay together and will not spread. Many tumors metastasize, which means some of the abnormal cells break off and enter the blood stream or lymph vessels, permitting them to travel to another location in the body. Once there, they continue reproducing furiously. Additional tumors form in these new sites, making treatment very difficult.

Normally the body recognizes damaged cells and immediately calls in protective forces to correct the situation before the reproduction of abnormal cells escalates out of hand. But cancer cells produce proteins which block the immune system from recognizing them. They even recruit the immune system to help them metastasize. Some scientists and a great deal of the lay public believe stress plays a role in cancer, suppressing the immune system so the body has trouble recognizing glitches and repairing them. The National Cancer Institute acknowledges psychological stress may play a role in the transformation of normal cells into cancerous cells, but more research is needed.[5]

Simple diet and lifestyle changes that reduce emotional and oxidative stress to the body can significantly reduce your cancer risk. According to the American Cancer Society, "Scientific evidence suggests that about one-third of the 571,950 cancer deaths expected to occur in 2011 will be related to overweight or obesity, physical inactivity, and nutrition and thus could also be prevented."[6]

## Honey Reduces Radiation Side Effects

As part of the treatment strategy to stop cancer, around 60 percent of all patients receive radiation treatment. Cancer cells replicate faster than healthy cells, so radiation therapy attempts to stop cancer by killing fast reproducing cells.

Using the focused energy of x-rays, gamma rays or other charged particles, radiation reacts with the water in cells and indirectly damages the genetic material that controls cell growth. Healthy cells can usually repair the damage, while cancerous cells cannot and so they die.

Since the radiation targets quickly reproducing cells, it also kills off the fast reproducing cells lining the entire gastrointestinal (GI) tract from the mouth to the anus. When these beneficial cells die along with cancerous material, it can lead to mucositis, the medical term for agonizing sores that develop along the complete length of the GI tract. They start as small whitish patches. By the third to sixth week of radiation therapy, the mouth and throat are raw and the large open sores bleed. Radiation creates an imbalance - more cells die along the GI tract than the body replenishes.

Large ulcers then develop, making it difficult to eat, drink or swallow. According to Dr. Biswa Biswal, from the Department of Nuclear Medicine, Radiotherapy and Oncology at University Sains in Malaysia, patients can no longer taste the food, as the radiation alters their taste buds.[7] When the ulcers become too painful, patients can't eat or drink.

They rapidly lose weight and often cease radiation, unable to bear the agonizing side effects.

"There is no established treatment available for this common problem," Dr. Biswal explained in an interview. "Thousands of head and neck cancer patients world-wide suffer from mucositis every day."

Dr. Biswal wanted to learn if honey could reduce some of the nasty side effects of radiation treatment. Every year doctors diagnose over 500,000 people worldwide with a form of head and neck cancer and treatment typically includes radiation therapy. In Dr. Biswal's clinical study, 40 patients with cancer in the neck and head region, such as mouth, throat or thyroid, were split evenly into two groups. [8] The first group received 20 ml (four teaspoons of honey) 15 minutes before their radiation treatment, a second dose 15 minutes after radiation and a final dose six hours post treatment. The patients were advised to swish the honey around their mouth first and then swallow slowly so it would coat the throat. The other group of 20 patients underwent the same type of radiation treatment, but without consuming any honey.

Dr. Biswal used honey gathered predominantly from the tea plant *Camellia sinensis*, which grows near the Cameron Highlands of Malaysia. The honey was filtered, but otherwise unprocessed. When bacteria inhabit the moist environment of the mouth, they aggravate the severity of mucositis and release toxins that cause oral inflammation.[9] Laboratory tests confirmed the honey was active against a range of common bacteria.

The honey group suffered significantly less mucositis. More than 75 percent of the 20 patients not taking honey suffered level three and four lesions; the most excruciating ulcerations. No one in the honey group had the painful mouth sores of the highest level and only 20 percent suffered from level three sores. Simple consumption of honey significantly reduced the pain level. Coating a wound with honey seals the damaged tissue from air and thus slows down tissue oxygenation. "This could dampen pain within 30 seconds after application," Dr. Biswal said.[10]

None of the honey consuming patients had to interrupt their radiation therapy. Four of the control patients developed such severe mouth ulceration they had to cease taking treatments for four to nine days. To reduce the pain, Dr. Biswal gave them topical anesthetics. Unable to eat or drink, the four individuals were hooked up to IV drips to supplement their nutrition.

Honey had an additional benefit. It helped stave off weight loss; a common occurrence that further weakens cancer patients. Fifty-five percent of those taking honey maintained or increased their body weight, compared to 25 percent in the control group. The majority of the 20 patients who did not receive honey lost weight. Most patients typically lose 10 kg (22 lbs) while undergoing radiation therapy, Dr. Biswal said.[11]

When ingested, honey acts as a soothing demulcent in the throat. The anti-inflammatory properties of honey reduce incidences of mucositis, helping to stem the nasty side effects of radiation before they become painful. Honey supports tissue regeneration in healthy cells, so any lost mucosal lining can quickly be replaced. Honey repairs tissues, controls pain, functions as a nutritional supplement and inhibits inflammation, said Dr. Biswal. "Easily available, cost-effective and …accessible to rich and poor alike, (honey is) an ideal option for radiation induced mucositis."[12]

"Honey could be the most cost effective treatment for radiation mucositis," Dr. Biswal said. Since honey proves so effective against radiation mucositis, it may also be effective in alleviating oral pain arising during chemotherapy treatments and the mucositis that develops in bone marrow transplant patients. "Perhaps," Dr. Biswal said, "honey could be …routine practice in the future."[13]

## Honey And Sexual Libido

Dr. Biswal also mentioned that several of the male patients reported an increased libido. The researchers could not explain why this occurred. "Perhaps honey might have aphrodisiac qualities,"[14] Dr. Biswal postulated.

Charles Butler, who in 1609 dedicated his book *The Feminine Monarchie* to the recently deceased Queen Elizabeth I, would agree. In addition to finally putting to rest the falsehood that a king ruled a beehive instead of a single queen, Butler mentioned honey aroused sexual desire.[15]

## Iran Repeats Radiation Results

A team of cancer researchers and dental specialists teamed up in Balbol, Iran to repeat a similar trial in the Balbolsar Center for Cancer.[16] The team led by two female doctors wanted to see how effective honey was against radiation induced mucositis. This time the trial was double-blinded, so neither the patients nor the doctors evaluating their progress knew which treatment an individual received, a process which increases the reliability of the results.

All of the 40 individuals recruited for the study suffered from head and neck cancer and received radiation therapy once a day, five days a week. The radiation therapy was repeated for five to seven weeks, depending on tumor severity. The doctors split them evenly into two groups. The first group consumed 20 ml of pure natural honey made from thyme and astragale in the Alborz Mountains of northern Iran 15 minutes prior, 15 minutes post and six hours after radiotherapy, while the control group rinsed with 20 ml of normal saline.

Laboratory tests revealed the Iranian honey was ineffective in inhibiting of variety of bacteria within 24 hours. Yet even without antibacterial activity, the honey proved very effective in mitigating mucositis.

The cancer patients consuming honey experienced significantly fewer mouth ulcerations and inflammation throughout the entire trial. Six individuals in the control group required medication to ease the pain of their severe mucositis, while none in the honey group needed such intervention. Three of the cancer patients who did not receive the honey therapy temporarily refused to continue treatment due to the pain in their mouths.

While the group rinsing with normal saline lost an average of 6.3 kg (13.9 lbs) during their cancer therapy, the honey group remained relatively stable, losing on average only one kilogram (2.2 lbs). Severe weight loss and anemia are common side effects of radiation therapy, putting additional stress on the body.

The team of doctors concluded: "Natural honey is a product with rich nutritional qualities that could be a pleasant, simple, and economic (solution) for the management of radiation mucositis."[17]

## Honey Protects Against Tooth Decay in Cancer Patients

Radiation therapy for head and neck cancer causes temporary or permanent damage to the glands that produce the mouth's saliva. Cancer patients commonly suffer from dry mouth. These changes affect the bacterial residents of the mouth and promote the development of tooth cavities. Most dental cavities are caused by the bacteria *Streptococcus mutans*, especially in cancer patients. Unheated honey stored out of the light to protect the glucose oxidase activity typically halts the growth of this destructive dental bacterium.

In a small clinical trial conducted in Israel, researchers found that swishing a wildflower honey in the mouth for five minutes significantly reduced the amount of *Streptococcus mutans* living in the mouths of cancer patients.[18] Another small trial found that honey does not erode tooth enamel in cancer patients, suggesting it can be safely consumed to combat the side effects of mucositis.[19]

## WHITE BLOOD CELL LIMBO: ACUTE FEBRILE NEUTROPENIA

Bone marrow, soft tissue hidden inside the hollows of our bones, produces immature, undifferentiated cells known as stem cells. These stem cells have the ability to develop into a large variety of different cell types, including red and white blood cells. The red blood cells transport oxygen throughout the body, keeping our tissues and organs functioning. The white blood cells ingest bacteria, debris and toxins, helping us fight infections.

Both radiation and chemotherapy attack fast reproducing cells, including the vital stem cells in our bone marrow. Without enough white blood cells circulating in our body, our immune system becomes depressed and we become prone to disease and infection. Normal adults average about 1,500 neutrophils per cubic millimeter of blood - a specific type of white blood cell that stops bacteria attacking the immune system. So long as you have more than 1,000, you have a normal level of protection against infection.

Should the neutrophils dip below 1,000, your immune system no longer functions well, leaving you susceptible to severe infection. If levels drop below 200, your immune system has quit working. At these dangerously low levels, you will be hospitalized and pumped full of antibiotics. Otherwise even normally benign infections become deadly.

By killing off rapidly reproducing cells, chemotherapy significantly reduces the blood cell production of bone marrow. This toxic side effect limits the amount of drugs an individual can withstand. Doctors have found that approximately seven to 14 days after a patient receives a chemotherapy cocktail, their neutrophil counts drop dramatically.

Without protective white blood cells to stave off infections, patients can develop acute febrile neutropenia. The long-winded medical name means a rapid onset of fever due to lack of neutrophils - a life threatening condition. Patients are immediately hospitalized and receive antibiotic injections directly into the bloodstream.

The cells that line our blood vessels produce a hormone which encourages our bone marrow to churn out white blood cells. Cancer patients receive injections of colony stimulating factor; a man-made version of this hormone to avoid recurrences of acute febrile neutropenia to help speed recovery. Currently injections add around $3,000 to the cost of medical care.

In a trial in Israel, 30 cancer patients had previously suffered from severe bouts of neutropenia, where their neutrophil counts dropped below 500.[20] Normally they would have received expensive colony stimulating factors for their second round of chemotherapy. Instead, they received five grams per day of Life-Mel honey on an empty stomach when they started the second bout of chemotherapy. Life-Mel honey is a natural honey made by bees foraging on medicinal plants, including:

*Echinacea pallidum*: pale purple coneflower
*Taraxacum officinalis*: dandelion
*Uncaria tomentosa*: cat's claw
*Chicorium intubus*: chicory
*Eleutherococcus senticosus*: Siberian ginseng
*Vaccinium myrtillis*: whortleberry or bilberry
*Urtica dioica*: stinging nettle
*Avena sativa*: oat
*Calendula officinalis*: marigold
*Inula helenium*: elecampane
*Trifolium pratense*: red clover
*Melilotus officinalis*: sweet, yellow clover
*Mellisa officinalis*: lemon balm
*Ficus carica*: fig
*Morus albus*: white mulberry
*Beta vulgaris*: beet
*Ribes rubrum*: red currant

For the five days of chemotherapy the 30 individuals consumed daily doses of honey. Although all of these patients had previously suffered from neutropenia when undergoing chemotherapy, 40 percent did not experience recurrences simply by taking the honey. One third of the patients felt they enjoyed an improved quality of life while consuming the honey.

Many people undergoing chemotherapy also experience anemia; a drop in red blood cells. Since chemotherapy kills off the rapidly reproducing stem cells in bone marrow, red blood cell production plummets. Yet we need red blood cells to deliver oxygen to our tissues and organs. The intake of honey reduced the occurrence of anemia in 64 percent of the patients without any negative side effects.

## Honey for Pediatric Cancer Patients

Over 90 percent of Dr. Simon's young patients at the pediatric oncology clinic at the University Clinic in Bonn undergo complex chemotherapy that involves five to six separate substances. Most of the children suffer from leukemia, brain tumors, and bone cancer. Due to the intensive chemical treatments, they have difficulties with wound healing and frequently experience amputations. Since lymphomas are highly malignant, doctors need to fight them with a stringent schedule of meds. Patients typically receive chemo for one week then they have three short weeks to recover before the whole process starts again. If doctors avoid resumption of chemo due to non-healing wounds, the child is prone to relapse.

Toni had a relapse of acute myeloid leukemia, a rare disease where the body produces too many white blood cells that never mature. These immature white blood cells build up in the bone marrow and prevent it from making healthy blood cells. After filling up the bone marrow, these improperly functioning white blood cells spill over into the blood stream. Toni developed a wound infection, but received allocation for a bone marrow transplantation from a donor with a close tissue match.

The transplantation had to be put on hold until the infection cleared, as Dr. Simon did not want to risk spreading the malevolent bacteria during the operation. By implementing Medihoney, a medical grade active honey, the infection disappeared. Toni continued to receive Medihoney applications during and after the transplant, leading to a successful conclusion.

Some of the parents of Dr. Simon's young patients were skeptical at first about the benefits of honey, but Dr. Simon was quick to point out that there were no sound arguments for other conventional treatments such as silver dressings. Little research has been done on the long-term effects of these conventional treatments which might negatively affect the development of young children.

Another common treatment is povidone-iodine, which "has the advantage of antiseptic properties and is well suited for skin disinfection prior to invasive procedures. However, we have decided against its use in wound care for our patients due to the adverse effects of systemic absorption of iodine on thyroid function."[21]

Dr. Simon explained, "These long term problems can be very detrimental. Thyroid function is suppressed by the transcutaneous (through the skin) uptake of iodine in newborn patients. In principle, the same problem exists with alcohol containing antiseptics, since they are almost completely absorbed and need to be metabolized by the children, who are receiving many other medications."[22] We really don't know enough about the long term effects of many commonly prescribed antibiotics on young children. In contrast, the natural substance honey does not display the problem of systemic absorption. Since the body does not absorb the honey, even patients with diabetes can safely apply honey to their wounds.

When Dr. Simon explained the successful results obtained through the application of Medihoney, the guardians of his young patients were usually eager to try the new approach. Because Medihoney is a convenient treatment, patients have responded very favorably. The honey keeps a moist, clean environment around the wound, so dry scabs do not form, turning normally agonizing dressing changes into a painless routine.

Doctors have known for a long time that moist environments benefit wound healing, but frequently avoid the situation as it encourages bacterial growth. Antimicrobial honey provides the ideal setting, inhibiting the growth of microbes while simultaneously permitting the wound to heal without forming dry scabs.

"Among other effects, honey stimulates the secretion of cytokines,"[23] which motivate and coordinate the process of inflammation and healing. Chronic wounds tend to smell foul, an embarrassing situation for a young child. Thankfully, honey treatments eliminate odor within days.

## Honey Heals Breast Cancer Skin Damage

The focused energy of radiation therapy damages the skin of most women undergoing radiation therapy for breast cancer. Typically it only causes redness, but in up to 20 percent it can cause more severe wounds. A team of doctors in the Netherlands recruited women whose skin could not withstand the onslaught of breast cancer radiation.[24] Of the 600 women receiving radiation therapy for their breast cancer, only twenty-seven experienced severe skin damage of grade three or higher.

Twenty-one women with 24 skin reactions agreed to participate in a trial to compare the effects of honey and paraffin dressings. Twelve of the wounds were treated with honey impregnated gauze dressings called HoneySoft, while the other twelve received conventional paraffin dressings.

With such a small trial, it is difficult to achieve statistically significant results. Yet the doctors noted a trend toward improved healing with honey. The twelve open wounds treated with honey closed, on average, in 11.9 compared to 13.9 days for the paraffin treated wounds. The skin completely healed within 18.4 days with the honey gauze versus 19.8 days for the paraffin. The women commented that the honey dressings reduced their pain and alleviated itching and irritation.

The doctors noted "greater patient satisfaction with honey than with paraffin" and concluded: "The use of honey gauze can be considered for the treatment of radiotherapy-induced dermatitis."[25]

A similar study recently conducted by Dr. Nichola Naidoo from the Waikato District Health Board in Hamilton, New Zealand compared pure active manuka honey to standard cream.[26] Eighty-one women undergoing radiation therapy for breast cancer received twice daily applications of manuka honey or cream to help reduce the incidence of skin damage - what doctors call radiation dermatitis. Thirty to 50 percent of all women undergoing breast cancer radiotherapy normally develop grade two skin damage.

The women applied the honey or cream twice daily, starting on the first day of radiation therapy and continued until ten days after they received their last radiation exposure. Just over one-third (37.2 percent) of the women using honey developed grade two or higher skin damage compared to more than half (57.8 percent) using the standard cream.

## Tumor Implantation

When doctors operate to remove cancer, there is always a risk of "seeding" a new tumor. The surgical intervention can accidentally spread a few cancerous cells, which then grow into a new tumor. Surgeons try to avoid disseminating cancerous cells in the operating zone or the blood stream.

Tumor implantation has become a concern in minimal invasive surgery, known as laparoscopic surgery, where doctors make only a tiny incision. They then insert plastic tubes, called ports. A minute video camera and several thin instruments are fed through these ports, so that the surgeon can see and operate.

There are many benefits to this technique, as the smaller incision results in smaller scars. The patient recovers faster and so spends less time in the hospital, returning to normal activities sooner. Unfortunately, this type of surgery has been linked to increased incidences of tumor implantation. Estimates show that approximately one to two percent of patients develop tumors from this type of surgery.[27]

A group of medical doctors in Istanbul, Turkey thought that a thin layer of honey covering the wound might provide protection against accidental tumor implantation. It would form a "tender film barrier, which could inhibit the attachment of tumor cells to the wound".[28]

They decided to test their theory in an animal study conducted in 2000 on tumor implantation in 60 mice.[29] The surgeons created wounds beneath the surface of the animals' skin. Half of the mice had honey applied to those wounds before and after their wounds were seeded with tumors. The other thirty mice served as the control group. The doctors also inoculated their wounds with tumors, but applied no honey.

All thirty of the second group, but only eight in the honey group, developed tumors. Simple application of honey to the wound before and after the tumor seeding stopped them from adhering and taking up residence in the majority of mice. Tumors that did develop in the honey treated mice were much smaller. The researchers surmised that the honey protected the wounds against tumor implantation by creating a protective barrier. A medical reviewer notes that the honey may have killed the tumor cells by dehydrating them and concludes: "The honey was well tolerated and could be considered for coating a trocar (a sharp surgical instrument used in laparoscopic surgery) to avoid tumor implantation."[30]

To properly supply medical care, small incisions into the body are often necessary. Such ports offer easy entry points for bacterial infections. Honey coatings have proven an effective strategy for reducing bacterial infections on catheter ports.[31] Because of honey's antimicrobial properties it helps to create and retain a sterile environment.

## BLADDER CANCER

Every year, doctors diagnose over 52,000 men and 18,000 women with bladder cancer.[32] By the time bladder cancer is discovered, most individuals have celebrated their 70th birthday. Much more common in men, especially smokers, bladder cancer often causes pain during urination. Some will see blood in their urine, spurring them to seek medical attention. Other common symptoms include an increase in the frequency of urination and feeling pressure to urinate, but then not needing to pee.

A team of researchers in Japan decided to test honey's ability to stop bladder cancer cells from replicating both in a petri dish and in an animal model.[33] Normal human cells have 46 chromosomes, the long thread like strands of genetic material. We inherit 23 chromosomes from each of our parents. Cancer cells frequently don't conform to this pattern; they can be short some chromosomes and have extra copies of others - a condition called aneuploidy.

The team in Japan noticed that the aneuploid cells disappeared when they added honey, while the cells with normal chromosome numbers remained alive. This suggests that honey may have "a specific effect against the more aggressive tumor cells", the doctors said.[34]

To see if honey proved effective outside of a petri dish, the team injected bladder cancer cells into mice. Once the tumor grew to 100-150 mm$^3$, the mice were divided into five different groups. Two of the groups received honey injections of 12 percent or six percent honey directly into the cancerous lesion. A third group had access to honey diluted by an equal volume of water for six hours every other day. The last two groups served as controls; one received saline injections while the other received no treatment at all.

Both the honey injections and the mice that drank honey water had significantly smaller tumors. Honey thus slowed the growth of already established tumors. While early evidence from animal trials has little practical value for medical interventions in humans, such preliminary evidence should spur further research into honey's anti-tumor effects.

## Honey in the Battle Against Cancer

More clinical trials are obviously needed to confirm the effectiveness of honey, but since honey is a perfectly safe food with no negative side effects, it seems people undergoing radiation and chemotherapy can benefit from this sweet spoonful of medicine to alleviate the nasty side effects of cancer treatment.

Patients and doctors may also want to consider applying honey to any incision sites to avoid tumor implantation and bacterial infections.

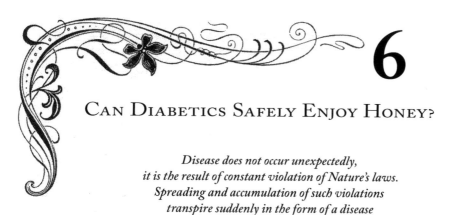

# 6

## Can Diabetics Safely Enjoy Honey?

*Disease does not occur unexpectedly,*
*it is the result of constant violation of Nature's laws.*
*Spreading and accumulation of such violations*
*transpire suddenly in the form of a disease*
*– but it only seems sudden.*

- Hippocrates

*In* recent years the number of Americans diagnosed with diabetes has skyrocketed, reaching epidemic proportions. All together one out of every twelve Americans has diabetes, a whopping 8.3 percent. While 18.8 million people know they suffer from this disease because they have been diagnosed, seven million individuals don't have a clue as they have not been diagnosed.[1]

If you discount children and only look at Americans that are at least 20 years old, the rate of diabetes climbs to 11.3 percent. More than one out of every 10 Americans old enough to purchase alcohol is diabetic. At current levels, if you make it to 65 years, you have slightly less than a one in four chance of being diabetic. Unfortunately the rate of diabetes continues to increase yearly. In 2010 alone 1.9 million new cases of diabetes were diagnosed. [2]

We all know that diabetes significantly affects a person's health. It is the seventh most common cause of death according to death certificates. However, since diabetes leads to a large range of complications—kidney failure, lower limb amputations, blindness, heart disease and stroke—it is only listed appropriately as the cause of death 10-15 percent of the time. According to Dr. Baer, a research physiologist with the USDA who spoke at the first International Symposium on Honey and Human Health, "That number is probably an underestimate. Most likely (diabetes) is the fourth or fifth most common killer, the leader being cardiovascular disease, followed by cancer."[3] A diabetic is twice as likely to die as a non-diabetic.[4]

Diabetes has been with us for a long time. The disease was first described as polyuria in the Egyptian Ebers Papyrus written around 1550 BC. Today 25.8 million people in the U.S. suffer from diabetes. When you add the 79 million pre-diabetics living in America, the rapid escalation of this disease is alarming.[5]

In the past doctors differentiated between juvenile and adult onset diabetes. More and more young children are now diagnosed with the type of diabetes previously only found in adults. Faced with misleading names, the medical community renamed juvenile and adult diabetes into type 1 and 2 diabetes respectively. Type 1 diabetes typically involves immune system issues that keep the pancreas from churning out enough insulin. In contrast, a person with type 2 diabetes often produces insulin, but the body no longer responds.

## Type 1 Diabetes

Previously called juvenile-onset diabetes or insulin-dependent diabetes mellitus, type 1 diabetics are unable to produce insulin. For some reason, the body's immune system views the normal and healthy production of beta cells in the pancreas as an invasion and so unleashes enzymes to destroy them. Pancreatic beta cells are the only cells in the entire body that can produce the regulatory hormone insulin.

When we eat a meal, the body breaks down the sugars and starches into glucose - the basic fuel that feeds all the cells of your body. Insulin takes the glucose circulating in the blood and pulls it into individual cells, where it is stored for later use to feed the brain and fuel basic body functions. Insulin regulates blood glucose levels, making sure they stay stable.

Without insulin injections, type 1 diabetics can't survive. Only through insulin injections or insulin pumps can they harvest and store energy from the food they eat. Insulin must be injected into the fat tissue beneath the skin. Unfortunately type 1 diabetics can't simply consume insulin, as stomach acid would break down the hormone just as it breaks down food.

According to the National Institute of Health, anywhere from five to 10 percent of all diabetics have type 1 diabetes. Risk factors for developing the disease may be related to autoimmune deficiencies, genetic or environmental influences.[6] Most frequently this type of diabetes strikes children and young adults. Currently there is no way to prevent or cure type 1 diabetes. Several clinical trials investigating methods of prevention are underway.

## PRE-DIABETES AND TYPE 2 DIABETES

Before individuals develop full-blown type 2 diabetes—previously known as adult-onset diabetes or non-insulin-dependent diabetes mellitus—they first become insulin resistant. In this pre-diabetic stage, the body still produces insulin, but the cells do not use it appropriately and so the glucose circulates in the blood instead of being stored for later use.

Because insulin no longer functions as it should, prediabetics have elevated levels of blood glucose, also known as hyperglycemia. A simple test performed after a night fast can determine if you are pre-diabetic.

Most prediabetics carry extra weight. The additional fat makes it more difficult for the body to use insulin correctly. But type 2 diabetes also develops in thin individuals, typically in the elderly.

By changing their diet, losing weight and exercising moderately every day, prediabetics can prevent or delay the onset of type 2 diabetes.[7] Since the body is no longer using insulin correctly, it requires more insulin to achieve the same effect. The pancreas tries to provide larger doses of insulin, churning it out in ever greater amounts. Eventually it simply can't keep up and loses its ability to produce insulin.

Glucose circulating in the blood starves cells of the energy they need to function. Over time continuously high blood glucose levels cause serious health issues; diabetics can go blind, experience kidney failure, and develop heart trouble.

## ESCALATING EPIDEMIC

"The rate of diabetes skyrocketed in the 1990s," research physiologist Dr. Baer from the USDA said, pointing to a bar chart on the screen behind him during the first International Symposium on Honey and Human Health.[8] "Before then it was fairly flat and stable at approximately six million people." The rate has since more than tripled.

Currently 35 percent of all Americans over twenty years of age are prediabetics.[9] Type 2 diabetes—previously an adult disease—has started to appear in young children and adolescents. While still rare, American Indians, African Americans, and Hispanic/Latino Americans are particularly at risk.[10] One out of every four obese children between the ages of four and 10 was pre-diabetic, researchers discovered in a clinical trial conducted in 2002. In obese adolescents between 11 and 18 years, 21 percent had elevated blood glucose levels indicative of pre-diabetes.[11]

Referring to a study in the *Journal of Medicinal Food*, Dr. Baer said all glucose resistant (pre-diabetics) and diabetics showed a favorable response to honey in comparison to glucose.[12] Compared to sugar, honey caused significantly lower blood glucose levels. Although honey caused an initial spike in blood glucose levels during the first half hour, these quickly subsided and honey resulted in lower blood glucose levels than sugar after 60, 120 and 180 minutes.

Other clinical trials have also demonstrated that honey does not raise blood glucose levels to the same extent as sucrose.[13,14] In a study involving 33 healthy individuals given a large dose of honey, sucrose or fructose (75 g) the researchers conclude: "Given that honey has a gentler effect on blood sugar levels on a per gram basis, and tastes sweeter than sucrose so that fewer grams would be consumed, it would seem prudent to recommend honey over sucrose."[15]

In a trial involving eight type 1 diabetics and six type 2 diabetics, honey again resulted in a lower glycemic response compared to sucrose or glucose. "We suggest that honey may prove to be a valuable sugar substitute in diabetics,"[16] the researchers concluded.

Dr. Baer believes the low glycemic index fructose content of honey, as well as the other minor sugar components, play an important role in glucose metabolism. "It might be worth looking at these minor constituents in greater detail," he said.[17]

Interestingly one clinical trial comparing the effect of honey and fructose in type 2 diabetics discovered that honey caused a much smaller spike in blood glucose levels than fructose.[18] The increase after glucose was

100 percent and fructose 81.3 percent, while honey resulted in a minimal increase of 32.4 percent. Based on the results of this trial, more than just the fructose content of honey must play a role in minimizing the effect on blood sugar levels. Why else would honey produce a lower rise than fructose?

## So Much More than Sugar Water

Honey contains low total antioxidants in comparison to other products such as berries. Yet surprisingly, *in vivo* tests indicate the body metabolizes and absorbs the antioxidants from honey mixed with water extremely well, which may make honey more effective than other foods with greater amounts of antioxidants.[19]

Many doctors and nutritionists mistakenly believe honey is nothing more than sugar water. "Honey is so much more," explains Dr. May Berenbaum, a phytochemist at the University of Illinois, who studies plant secretions.[20] "Nectar, as a plant tissue, is full of biologically active substances. It really bothers me when it's just called sugar water." Her research and that of her colleagues clearly demonstrates honey contains much more than table sugar. Honey includes minerals and high levels of antioxidants, especially the darker honeys.[21]

"Roman legionnaires used honey in their medical kits. We seem destined to rediscover things," Dr. Berenbaum added with a hint of irony.[22] In the 1990s honey was frowned upon by many health nutritionists, but this ancient remedy is finally receiving its due recognition. "*Parade* magazine just listed honey as one of the six super foods you should know about," Dr. Berenbaum said.

As Dr. Baer suggested, perhaps the combination of these trace elements and other sugar components positively influence blood sugar levels after honey consumption.

## Nectar Source Matters

Not all honeys are created equally. Honey is predominantly a glucose and fructose solution, but most people are unaware that the sugar ratios vary depending on the nectar source. Some honeys have less glucose content and more fructose. Since fructose is a lower GI food than glucose, many believe these low glucose honeys can be better tolerated by diabetics. These include black locust (*Robinia pseudoacacia*), sweet chestnut, and fir honey. Unfortunately the last two varieties are not harvested in the U.S., but can be found in some specialty shops that import honey from

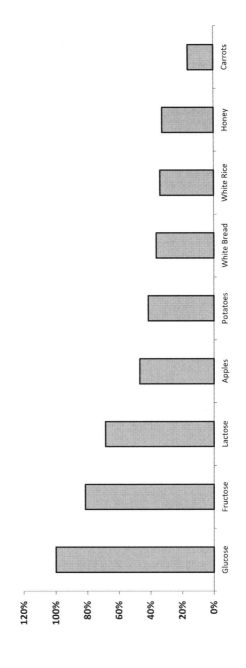

Blood Glucose Levels after Consuming Various Foods

Europe where they have still have large forests of sweet chestnut and fir trees.

As mentioned above, a clinical study comparing a variety of sugar types and other food products found [23] honey elicits a lower increase in blood sugar than fructose. Participants were given the same quantity of carbohydrates (25 grams) from each of nine different substances. This caused the actual serving size of the different foods to vary considerably, as some are more carbohydrate rich than others.

One 30 g serving of honey produced a lower rise in blood glucose levels (32.4 percent) than 25 g of glucose (100 percent), fructose (81.3 percent), or lactose (68.6 percent). Honey produced a smaller spike than 150 g serving of apples (46.9 percent), 125 g of potatoes (41.4 percent), 50 g of white bread (36.3 percent), and 125 g of white rice (33.8 percent). Only a serving of 260 g of carrots produced a lower blood glucose response (16.1 percent) than honey. (See table on left.)

## LIQUID GOLD

If there are more than 32 g of glucose per 100 g of honey, the high glucose concentration causes the honey to crystallize. In contrast, honey with less than 32 g of glucose will stay fluid for long periods of time. Since most consumers in the United States are only familiar with liquid honey and do not purchase finely crystallized honey, honey packers and beekeepers often heat their honey to re-liquefy it. So just because a honey is liquid in the States, does not mean it has a low glucose content. Unfortunately this heating also destroys some of the health benefits of the honey.

In Germany, where honey may not be heated above 105° F, high glucose honey is sold in a finely crystallized state that is spreadable and won't run off your bread. Most European beekeepers can inform you whether a particular honey will crystallize. Honeys that crystallize contain more glucose and less fructose and so may be less well tolerated by diabetics. Black locust, chestnut, and thyme honey have a high fructose to glucose ratio, suggesting they would be well tolerated by diabetics.

## A SPOONFUL A DAY

Diabetics should still not overindulge in honey, as it is a carbohydrate. But I have spoken with many diabetics who enjoy a daily spoonful of honey without negative effects on their blood sugar levels.

## Glucose and Fructose Content in Varietal Honeys

| Honey Variety | Fructose (g/100 g) | Glucose (g/100 g) | Fruc.+Gluc. (g/100 g) | Fruc./Gluc. ratio |
|---|---|---|---|---|
| *Arbutus* Madrones | 37.6 ± 1.5 | 32.7 ± 1.2 | 70.3 ± 2.3 | 1.15 ± 0.05 |
| *Brassica* | 38.3 ± 1.7 | 40.5 ± 2.6 | 78.7 ± 3.5 | 0.95 ± 0.07 |
| *Calluna* Heather | 40.8 ± 2.0 | 32.5 ± 1.6 | 73.4 ± 3.1 | 1.26 ± 0.07 |
| *Castanea* Chestnut | 40.8 ± 2.6 | 27.9 ± 2.5 | 68.7 ± 2.5 | 1.48 ± 0.19 |
| *Citrus* Citrus | 38.7 ± 2.6 | 31.4 ± 2.1 | 70.1 ± 3.5 | 1.24 ± 0.12 |
| *Erica arborea* Tree heather | 38.4 ± 1.3 | 34.7 ± 1.2 | 73.1 ± 1.6 | 1.11 ± 0.06 |
| *Eucalyptus* Eucalyptus | 39.1 ± 2.2 | 33.0 ± 1.9 | 72.0 ± 3.3 | 1.19 ± 0.09 |
| *Hedysarum* Sweet vetch | 39.0 ± 1.4 | 32.1 ± 1.3 | 71.1 ± 1.9 | 1.22 ± 0.07 |
| *Helianthus* Sunflower | 39.2 ± 1.6 | 37.4 ± 1.5 | 76.7 ± 2.7 | 1.05 ± 0.04 |
| *Lavandula* Lavender | 36.0 ±1.9 | 30.6 ± 1.7 | 66.6 ± 2.9 | 1.18 ± 0.07 |
| *Phacelia* Phacelia | 37.3 ± 2.5 | 34.0 ± 1.9 | 71.3 ± 3.8 | 1.10 ± 0.08 |
| *Rhododendron* Rhododendron | 39.1 ± 2.1 | 30.4 ± 2.2 | 69.6 ± 3.4 | 1.29 ± 0.10 |
| *Robinia* Black locust | 42.7 ± 2.3 | 26.5 ± 1.7 | 69.2 ± 3.3 | 1.61 ± 0.11 |
| *Rosmarinus* Rosemary | 38.4 ± 1.6 | 33.1 ± 2.2 | 71.5 ± 3.0 | 1.16 ± 0.08 |
| *Taraxacum* Dandelion | 37.4 ± 1.8 | 38.0 ± 2.8 | 75.2 ± 3.9 | 0.99 ± 0.07 |
| *Thymus* Thyme | 42.4 ± 2.4 | 30.3 ± 1.8 | 72.7 ± 2.9 | 1.41 ± 0.12 |
| *Tilia* Linden/Basswood | 37.5 ± 2.9 | 31.9 ± 2.5 | 69.5 ± 4.0 | 1.18 ± 0.12 |
| Honeydew | 32.5 ± 1.9 | 26.2 ± 2.5 | 58.7 ± 3.8 | 1.25 ± 0.12 |
| *Metcalfa* honeydew | 31.6 ± 3.2 | 23.9 ± 2.7 | 55.5 ± 4.5 | 1.34 ± 0.18 |

Table reproduced from Persano Oddo, L. and R. Piro (2004). "Main European unifloral honeys: descriptive sheets." Apidologie 35: S38-S81.

A long term animal study suggests honey actually decreases blood glucose levels, called HbA1c. Doctors monitor this level in diabetics and at-risk individuals. The HbA1c levels testify to the amount of glucose that binds to hemoglobin proteins in the blood. The levels do not fluctuate widely, giving insight into blood sugar levels over the last six to twelve weeks. The HbA1c levels were significantly lower in the honey fed animal group than in the sucrose group, while the sugar free control animals fell in the middle.[24]

Preliminary research certainly indicates that honey is not just "sugar water". The other constituents of honey appear to positively affect how the body absorbs the sugars from honey. More research and larger clinical trials are needed to say for certain what doses a diabetic can safely consume. But the first results look very promising. Since all people, including diabetics, like an occasional sweet reward, honey many prove to be the ideal sweetener.

## WOUND CARE FOR DIABETICS

As discussed later in Part II, honey is an excellent product in wound care. Rich in antibacterial properties, honey has proven especially effective in treating chronic and infected diabetic ulcers. Sadly of the two million chronic diabetic foot ulcers in the United States, many eventually lead to amputation. The two year survival rate after an amputation is only 50-60 percent for diabetic patients.[25]

Diabetics and their primary care providers are typically unaware that honey may provide the perfect remedy. In June 2007 the FDA approved honey wound care dressings. These have been implemented successfully on numerous diabetic patients whose ulcers had been infected with super-bugs at the Georgetown University Hospital's Center for Wound Healing.

Diabetic ulcers are a form of chronic wound, which stall in the inflammatory stage of healing. They can be very difficult to treat using conventional therapies. In seven clinical trials involving 255 patients with chronic wounds, honey produced very positive results.[26]

Dr. Jennifer Eddy in Wisconsin has treated several diabetic foot ulcers successfully with regular store bought honey straight off the super-market shelf. Some diabetics falsely fear their sugar intolerance makes them unsuitable candidates for honey wound treatments. According to Dr. Arne Simon from the Pediatric Oncology Center at the University of Bonn Clinic in Germany, the honey placed on a wound is not systemically absorbed into the blood flow. Diabetics using honey wound care products have not shown insulin spikes or other negative side-effects.

Part of the reason diabetic wounds may heal so slowly could be due to their lack of insulin. Not only does insulin permit cells to pull in glucose, it also acts as a growth hormone. When doctors give diabetics intravenous infusions or topical applications of insulin, their wounds heal faster.[27,28,29]

Honey mimics the effects of insulin. When diabetics inhaled honey as an aerosol, it reduced blood glucose levels 30 minutes after inhalation, fasting blood glucose levels three hours later and significantly lowered hyperglycemia.[30]

While I was giving a talk on the health benefits of honey in Raleigh, North Carolina a woman approached my husband. Doctors had informed her 96-year-old mother that her foot would have to be removed due to chronic diabetic foot ulcers. Her mother told the doctors she preferred to self-treat her foot with honey. "They thought she was crazy, but it worked," the woman said. "She just didn't want to lose her foot."

One anecdotal story carries little weight in scientific circles. To date more than a hundred case studies and numerous clinical trials[31] confirm honey has an amazing potential to kick-start the healing process of chronic wounds, such as diabetic ulcers. If you or someone you know has been fighting with a diabetic ulcer, honey dressings could provide a sweet solution.

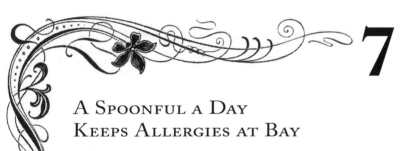

## A Spoonful a Day
## Keeps Allergies at Bay

*Hay fever is the most common allergy in the developed world.*
*Yet, there are some countries in the world*
*where doctors don't know what hay fever is.*

- Dr. Joel Weinstock,
Professor of Medicine and Immunology
Tufts University

*A*llergies caused by airborne pollen ruin one of the prettiest times of year for over 17 million Americans each year.[1] Ragweed hay fever afflicts 15 percent of all Americans.[2] Instead of enjoying the beauty of nature unfurling after winter, these individuals hide inside every spring to avoid runny noses, tearing eyes and constricted breathing brought on by the swirls of wind-borne pollen that fill the air. On any given day 10,000 children miss school because of hay fever, according to the American Academy of Allergy, Asthma and Immunology.[3]

Many desperate individuals seek medical help, splurging on over the counter allergy medicines, prescriptions or expensive desensitization therapy. Hay fever causes Americans to seek the help and advice of their medical doctor 16.7 million times every year - countless hours spent in waiting rooms, tissues clutched in hand, miserably awaiting some form of relief.

After years of suffering some decide to try desensitization. This therapy, which was invented in 1911 in St. Mary's Hospital in London, injects ever increasing amounts of the allergen into a patient. Desensitization therapy gradually builds up the body's immunity to the allergen. Unfortunately some individuals undergoing treatment suffer anaphylactic shock, a severe allergic reaction that causes a rapid pulse, constriction of the throat and a sudden drop in blood pressure. If not treated immediately, anaphylactic shock can prove fatal. A shot of adrenaline slows the body's reaction until appropriate medical care can be administered.

But before investing your hard earned money in desensitization, antihistamines and other remedies, why not see if honey bees can help? These hard working ladies gather nectar from a wide variety of plants. Most spring allergies are caused by the overabundance of wind-borne pollen. These ubiquitous miniscule grains also drift into the nectar of other plants, which the bees then gather and turn into honey.

Consuming a spoonful of *local* honey *every day*, preferably starting at least one month before spring, many believe helps desensitize your body to the pollen in your environment. Others insist chewing on the wax cappings beekeepers cut off when harvesting honey brings the greatest relief, as these contain more traces of pollen.

As far back as 1759, Sir John Hill, an authority on natural medicines, published a small work entitled *The Virtues of Honey*. During his lifetime, hay fever was believed to be a type of asthma. He describes how "by the use of honey alone this complaint will gradually wear off".[4]

The U.S. military has also noted the potential of honey to treat hay fever. Captain George D McGrew published a report in the *Transactions of the Association of Military Surgeons* entitled "Time and Money Saved in the Treatment of Hay Fever". He noted:

> *Among the many home remedies for the treatment of hay fever brought up in discussions with the afflicted, one alone seemed of real value. Several individuals state that, in the past year or two, they had received varying degrees of relief from symptoms by the eating of honey produced in their vicinity, and particularly from the chewing of comb*

*wax. It was reasonable to infer from this that the benefit received was probably from the oral extraction of the pollen in the honey and wax.[5]*

Anecdotal evidence for the use of honey to treat hay fever abounds, but so far medical researchers have not yet put honey to the test in a widespread clinical trial. However, in Britain Dr. Croft completed a small trial involving twenty-one patients.[6] All had suffered from hay fever for numerous years. Half of them had previously tried desensitization shots, but the treatment failed to produce long term results.

Dr. Croft decided it was nearly impossible to conduct a double-blind study with honey, since honey is so recognizable by its taste and aroma. Instead the participants were instructed to consume 10-20 grams of honey every day and report their symptoms. They started consuming honey prior to the start of hay fever season.

Sixteen of the participants (76 percent) reported improvement due to the honey consumption. Seven of those sixteen (44 percent) emphasized that the honey had been "a great benefit". One patient, who had suffered from hay fever for the last 27 years, noted that due to the honey they needed "no medication for hay fever was needed (as) in previous years".

Those who firmly believe in the effects of honey against hay fever tend to recommend local honey, since locally produced honey most likely contains minute traces of the specific allergens bothering you. A safe food consumed by millions of people around the world, honey may prove effective for you. (A few rare individuals are allergic to honey. If you notice any allergic symptoms after consuming honey, please seek appropriate medical attention).

If you decide to try honey for your allergies, stick with this sweet remedy for at least four to eight weeks, before you give up. It is believed that the pollen traces contained in the honey pass through the gut wall and then enter the blood stream. Here they come in contact with cells that form antibodies. By continually exposing the body to minute doses, the body has a chance to build up resistance. Naturally this takes time. But with all of the other health benefits attributed to honey, daily consumption should be a joy.

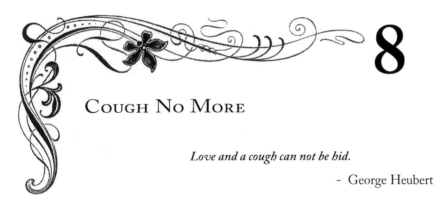

## COUGH NO MORE

*Love and a cough can not be hid.*

- George Heubert

$\mathcal{W}$hen you were little and showed the slightest hint of a cough, did your grandmother insist on a spoonful of honey or a small chunk of comb honey to help soothe your throat? She may have known best. A recent clinical trial at Penn State College of Medicine clearly showed honey was more effective at alleviating cough symptoms than over-the-counter cold medicines.[1]

I was surprised to learn that a cough is the most common symptom that leads us to seek out acute medical care. Many of us go to the doctor in the belief he will prescribe something to cure what ails us. Forty-four percent of Americans incorrectly assume antibiotics will cure the common cold.[2] So when our children start coughing, we tend to head straight to the doctor or the hospital. Eager to help their children, parents often pressure doctors to "do something" and don't understand an instant cure does not exist.[3]

According to Dr. Jessica Beiler, who presented research results on behalf of her colleague Dr. Ian Paul from Penn State Children's Hospital, we spend billions every year on over-the-counter cough and cold medicines. "Parents are naturally concerned about their child's health," Dr. Beiler said, emphasizing each word to highlight their importance. "Most common treatments are ineffective."[4]

The most frequently used cough suppressant is dextromethorphan (DM). However, when Dr. Ian Paul conducted a clinical trial in 2004, he discovered that DM and another type of active ingredient called diphenhydramine did not alleviate nocturnal cough or sleep difficulties in children suffering from upper respiratory infections any better than a placebo.[5] In fact the DM caused greater incidences of insomnia, while diphenhydramine caused drowsiness.

As far back as 1997 the American Academy of Pediatrics Committee on Drugs found there were no well controlled scientific studies that showed that DM was effective or safe for children.[6] A review of medical trials on chronic coughs in children found "no evidence for using medications for the symptomatic relief of cough".[7] It recommended over-the-counter medications be avoided, especially in young children, as they can cause illness and death.

In January 2007, the Center for Disease Control and Prevention reiterated the potential harm to young children when they published a report entitled "Infant Deaths Associated with Cough and Cold Medications" in their weekly MMRW report.[8] They noted that over 1,500 children under the age of two were treated in emergency rooms for adverse reactions to over-the-counter cough medicines in 2005. Three infants died due to the medication. Later that same year drug companies pulled their infant cough medicines from the shelves before the FDA met for an advisory committee meeting.

With so much potential harm in cough medicines, Dr. Ian Paul decided to look at safe alternatives. In 2001, the World Health Organization recommended honey as a safe demulcent that coats the throat and soothes irritated mucus membranes.[9] Honey, they concluded, was a cheap, popular and safe alternative to cough medicines for reducing cough and dry throat symptoms. The belief that honey helps alleviate coughs spans numerous cultures around the world as far away as Russia, Sri Lanka, India, Mexico and Germany, to name just a few.[10]

Dr. Paul and his colleagues designed a study to compare identical doses of buckwheat honey or honey flavored DM against a placebo to determine which would help reduce night time coughing and improve sleep quality in children aged two to 18 years.[11] One hundred and five children who had been ill for an average of 4.6 days before visiting the clinic participated in the trial. None of them had received cough medicine the night before. The children receiving the honey had reduced incidences of cough and slept better compared to the DM cough medicine and the placebo. The concerned parents also enjoyed a more restive night's sleep, knowing they had done something to help their offspring.

The FDA recently recommended parents not give DM cough medicine to children under the age of two and take extra caution with children younger than eleven.[12] Parents in these categories will most likely seek alternatives and honey certainly fits the bill. A potent anti-inflammatory, honey quickly soothes the throat. Honey's sweetness also acts as a demulcent, stimulating the secretion of saliva and reducing coughing fits. When your grandmother reached for that jar of honey, she really did know best. The antimicrobial and antioxidant properties of honey add to the beneficial effect.

One of the most frequent uses of honey in the United States is as an ingredient in cough drops. Before you grab a bag, be sure to read the fine print on the ingredient list. Most honey cough drops contain only minute amounts of honey; regular sugar or corn syrup being the predominant sweetener. Honey should be listed first before corn syrup, sucrose or any other type of sweetener to reap the full benefits of this natural remedy.

# *Interlude*

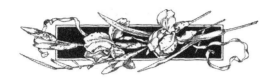

## *The Land of Milk and Honey*

When the Jews fled from Egypt, God promised to lead them into a land that flowed with milk and honey. Judging by the phrase "he made him to suck honey out of the rock" (Deuteronomy 32.13), feral hives of bees, which build their wild nests in cave openings, existed in abundance in the Promised Land. Man plundered the sweet bounty of wild combs filled with honey, winning a tasty and nutritious treat.

The tradition of enjoying honey persists in the Jewish religion to this day. On Rosh Hashanah, Jews toast the New Year with apple slices dipped in honey, representing the wish for a sweet new year.

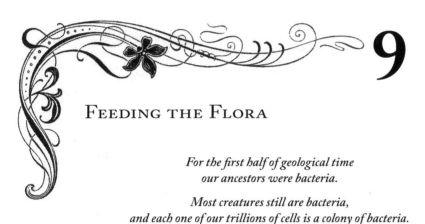

## FEEDING THE FLORA

*For the first half of geological time*
*our ancestors were bacteria.*

*Most creatures still are bacteria,*
*and each one of our trillions of cells is a colony of bacteria.*

- Richard Dawkins

*We* are full of bacteria. They live on us and in us, happily setting up camp on our skin, in our nose and intestines. Bacteria pervade our body, much like children romp through a school. A few limited places, like the teacher's lounge and adult restrooms, are off limits in schools. The same goes for our body. Under normal circumstances our blood, brain, urinary tract and lungs are sterile, as if bright yellow "do not enter" police tape blocked the way in for bacteria.

While we tend to think of ourselves as individuals, our bodies hold many more species than the average zoo. Five hundred to 100,000 different species of bacteria call our body home. Exceedingly small, around 1,000,000,000,000,000 bacteria ($10^{15}$) cram into a single human body.

These bacteria live unobtrusively, munching away on dead cells, nutrients and other elements.

A large majority colonize our digestive tract, where they attach to the wall, chewing on nutrients we can't break down ourselves. They've earned the pretty moniker gut flora, as if they were a vast array of flowers blooming along the twists and turns of our intestine. Although we enter the world without these cooperative microflora in our infant intestine, they start to take up residence within one week, where they form "a natural defense barrier against harmful microbes in the environment".[1] During our first year of life, the colonizing microflora remain unstable, but settle down by the time we celebrate our first birthday.[2]

These beneficial bacteria help digest our food, breaking down complex nutrients such as carbohydrates as they travel the long, winding route from stomach to anus. Just like plants, they compete for ground space with other species. By their presence, beneficial bacteria obstruct nasty, detrimental ones from adhering to their territory in the GI tract.

You've probably heard the terms prebiotics and probiotics bandied about when reading up on a healthy lifestyle and the secrets to good health. Or maybe the many commercials on television proclaiming the active ingredients in yogurt ring a bell. What *exactly* are probiotics and prebiotics?

Probiotics are defined as "living microorganisms, which on ingestion in sufficient numbers, exert health benefits beyond inherent basic nutrition".[3] Picture them as millions of tiny cowboys wearing big white hats, the good guys, live bacteria that defend the 30 feet of your intestine, with a surface area equivalent to a football field. Probiotics inhibit the growth of pathogens, reduce colon cancer risk, stimulate our immune system and reduce blood cholesterol levels[4] - quite a lot considering their miniscule size.

Currently identified probiotics are either lactic acid bacteria (lactobacilli) or bifidobacteria, but it's still a relatively new field of research, so more types may be discovered in the future. To live and fight, these hard working probiotics need sustenance. This is where prebiotics enter the picture. Prebiotics move undigested through the stomach and upper intestine into the lower intestine, where they promote the growth and activity of our white-hatted heroes.

Usually these prebiotics are oligosaccharides, carbohydrates composed of three or more simple sugars. Oligosaccharides make up only 4.2 percent of honey.[5] But Dr. Peter Molan, from the Honey Research Unit at

Waikato University in New Zealand, believes the excess fructose in most honeys passes undigested into the lower intestine, where it feeds these good bacteria and stimulates their rate of growth.[6]

Lab tests demonstrate that a five percent honey solution added to yogurt produces higher levels of bifidobacteria. It also stimulates acid production from bifidobacteria, which has been linked to numerous health benefits.[7, 8] Simply enjoying a regular spoonful of honey may support those beneficial bacterial inhabitants of your intestinal tract.

## HONEY THE PRO

A husband and wife team, Dr. Tobias Olofsson and Dr. Alejandro Vasquez from Lund, Sweden discovered fresh honey contains different types of probiotic lactic acid bacteria (LAB); beneficial bacteria similar to the ones that colonize our gastrointestinal tract. In their lab at the University of Sweden, they detected six types of lactobacillus and four types of bifidobacteria in the honey stomach of the honey bee and in fresh honey, whose moisture content was still above 22 percent.[9]

When beekeepers harvest honey, its moisture content typically doesn't exceed 18 percent, otherwise the honey contains enough water to allow the naturally occurring yeasts to ferment. Fermented honey was most likely the world's first alcoholic beverage. Through the Middle Ages, fermented honey wines called mead were the alcoholic beverage of choice for both noblemen and peasants. The original Queen Elizabeth loved metheglin, spiced mead; traditionally brewed with medicinal herbs, the name means "medicinal mead".

Once the bees dehydrate the honey to a low moisture content, turning it into a stable product that can be stored for years, the beneficial bacteria cannot survive in the super saturated sugar. Although they disappear, they leave behind useful compounds. Many components of honey, such as lactic acid, acetic acid, formic acid, hydrogen peroxide and bacteriocins may trace back to these beneficial organisms.[10]

According to the Swedish researchers, no one has previously discovered these beneficial bacteria in honey. Additional research must first be completed before a clearer picture can emerge, but the discovery of LAB in fresh honey is a significant find.

## LAND OF MILK AND HONEY

The Old Testament promised to deliver the Israelites into the land of milk and honey when they fled Egypt. The association between milk and honey survives in numerous cultures. The infamous seductress Cleopatra charmed two of the most powerful men with her beguiling ways. One of her beauty secrets: luxuriating in regular baths of milk and honey to retain her youthful appearance.

"A letter from the Grand Vizier of the Mongol Empire in about 1300 mentions a present of honey and yogurt; sweets of dried yogurt and honey are sold to this day in Central Asian markets."[11]

The wide spread use of dairy products combined with honey throughout the world indicates our ancestors observed the beneficial results without necessarily understanding why the combination worked so well. Modern researchers have now unraveled the secret: honey provides food for the beneficial bacteria, supporting their growth in fermented foods like yogurt and also in our intestine. As consumers demand more natural products, honey sweetened yogurt has become a staple in the grocery store.[12]

---

### Cleopatra's Secret to Great Skin

Enjoy Cleopatra's opulence by drizzling ½ cup of honey and 2-4 cups of fresh milk into a warm tub for a relaxing soak. Honey helps clean your skin, while the milk rejuvenates it, making your skin appear fresh and young.

Milk contains lactic acid, an alpha hydroxy acid, which exfoliates your skin by dissolving the glue like substance that keeps dead skin cells clumped together. The mild acid allows the dead skin to slough off, revealing healthy new skin below. Those seeking younger looking skin should protect themselves from the sun; alpha hydroxy treatments leave skin more sensitive to the damaging effects of ultra violet light.

---

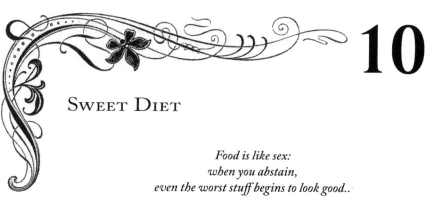

# 10

## SWEET DIET

*Food is like sex:*
*when you abstain,*
*even the worst stuff begins to look good..*

\- Beth McCollister

*One should eat to live,*
*not live to eat.*

\- Cicero,
Rhetoricorum LV

*To* avoid gaining weight, we often shun fatty foods. "Fat intake decreased over the last twenty years, but obesity increased," Dr. Nicola Starkey explained during her presentation at the First International Symposium on Honey and Human Health in Sacramento, CA.[1]

Obviously something isn't working out right, if we eat less fat yet are more obese. Dr. Starkey believes the key to this conundrum may lie in our high sugar consumption. She works as a behavioral psychologist at the Honey Research Unit, Waikato University, New Zealand. Along with her graduate student Lynne Chepulis, Starkey completed an animal study looking at the long term effects of a diet rich in honey or sugar.[2]

In our modern society, we fear putting on weight. Low fat foods now fill our supermarket shelves, appealing to our desire to stay slender. To make low fat diets palatable, they contain inordinate amounts of sugar. High sugar foods are usually high glycemic index (GI) foods, which flood our blood with glucose, causing a spike in insulin. Over time this overstimulation can lead to the development of type 2 diabetes.

High levels of blood glucose negatively impact our health. They cause oxidative stress, damaging our cells through free radicals. Antioxidants help counteract these destructive free radicals, but age decreases their production. "The brain is very susceptible," Dr. Starkey emphasized, "as it is the largest user of glucose. The free radicals attack our brain cells. There is a link between this oxidative stress and our thinking abilities, a link with Alzheimer's."[3]

A diet of low GI foods can improve our cognitive ability, especially our working memory that lets us analyze multiple things at the same time. Working memory springs into action every time we get behind the wheel of our car, letting us maneuver the car through traffic, alert to road signals and pedestrians. It also helps process and cement information from short term memory into long term memory.

Scores of primary physicians mistakenly believe honey to be the same as refined sugar. In fact honey is a relatively low GI food, although there is some variance from one type of honey to the next. Black locust honey earns the lowest GI score of 32, while the average GI score of all honey was 55, compared to 68 for sucrose.[4]

To see the long term effects of sugar consumption, Starkey and Chepulis studied animals that put on weight under stress, just like humans. They were divided into three groups: the control animals received a sugar-free diet, a second group was fed a diet with 7.9 percent sucrose and the last group a diet made with 10 percent honey. The honey fed group received a higher percentage than the sugar group to make up for honey's moisture content - this equalized their exposure to sweets. The animals could eat as much food as they wanted.

While the differences were not significant in the first few weeks, after 12 months the sucrose fed animals had gained 23 percent more weight than the animals on the honey or sugar-free diet, despite all three groups eating similar amounts of food. Twenty-three percent might not sound like a big deal, but it translates into substantial extra weight. By consuming sucrose instead of honey, the animals put on an extra one fifth of their total body weight. Converted into human terms, if you weighed 135 lbs before starting the diet, you would jump to 166 lbs after one year.

The researchers also measured HbA1c levels, which measures the amount of glycated hemoglobin in the blood. As explained previously, hemoglobin is a blood protein that shuttles oxygen. If your blood glucose levels have been very high in the last six to twelve weeks, sugars attach to hemoglobin and they become glycated. Doctors monitor HbA1c levels in diabetics and at-risk individuals to see how they have been keeping their blood glucose levels in check. Diabetics have rates above 6.5, while healthy individuals typically have levels around four.

In the New Zealand animal trial, after 12 months of the different diets, the HbA1c levels were significantly lower in honey (3.97) than sucrose (4.19) group, while the sugar free control animals had a rate of 4.07.[5]

## THE GOOD, THE BAD, AND THE UGLY

The scientists were surprised to find that honey also boosted good HDL cholesterol compared to the sucrose and sugar-free diet. High levels of HDL cholesterol protect against heart attacks. According to the American Heart Association "medical experts think that HDL tends to carry cholesterol away from the arteries and back to the liver, where it's passed from the body. Some experts believe that HDL removes excess cholesterol from arterial plaque, slowing its buildup."[6]

So high levels of HDL are more likely to protect you from a heart attack, while low levels make you more susceptible. A diet that includes honey instead of sucrose or sugar-free substitutes raised HDL levels in animals. The same may occur in humans, but the trials have not yet been carried out.

Most importantly, the honey fed animals showed less oxidative brain damage than the other two groups. In addition to measuring weight and blood glucose levels, the animals also underwent behavioral tests. The longer the animals stayed on the honey diet, the better their ability to remember mazes and the less anxiety they exhibited.

Since the honey diet caused less oxidative damage, Dr. Starkey theorized that perhaps honey protected the hippocampus in the brain, as this small part of the forebrain affects both anxiety and long-term memory. "It's extremely susceptible to oxidative damage," she explained. The first symptoms of a damaged hippocampus are memory problems and disorientation.

If humans react the same way to honey incorporated into the diet, eating for weight loss has never been sweeter. The next time you're craving something sweet, consider swapping out your table sugar for a jar of honey.

## The Skinny on Artificial Sweeteners

New research shows that artificial sweeteners confuse our brains.[7] Unlike real sugar, the artificial sweeteners trigger a weak pleasure response. Yet the pseudo sugars inspire greater communication between brain regions. Consumption of artificial sweeteners stimulates the reward region, but does not satiate it. Researchers believe this may be due to a poor feedback system, so that the craving for sweets is not squelched.

Artificial sweeteners may also throw off our internal calorie counter.[8,9] When we consume sugar-free foods, we stop associating sweetness with calories and so tend to over eat. Overindulging leads to weight gain and obesity. These same artificial sweeteners seem to slow down our metabolism, so that we have a harder time shedding extra pounds.

Honey could provide the perfect solution. Composed of true sugars, it would satisfy our cravings for sweets, but may not lead to putting on pounds. As mentioned previously, it is easy to munch through an entire chocolate bar in a single sitting. You would be hard pressed to consume the same volume of honey in one go. Why not try it yourself the next time you crave something sweet. I bet you'll notice after a few spoonfuls of honey, you're full.

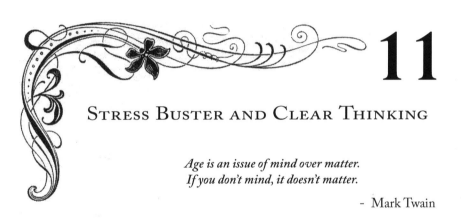

# 11

## STRESS BUSTER AND CLEAR THINKING

*Age is an issue of mind over matter.*
*If you don't mind, it doesn't matter.*

- Mark Twain

*O*ur bodies start to break down with time. As mentioned in the chapter on honey as an ideal food, one scientist describes aging as the body slowly going rancid. Our immune system responses decline as we age. Scientists believe this slower immune response is linked to a reduction in a specific type of white blood cell called a lymphocyte.[1] These small white blood cells play a crucial role in defending our bodies against invaders.

### REVERSING THE CLOCK

There are two types of lymphocytes called T cells and B cells. The T cells earned their name because they mature in the thymus gland. They do a lot of the grunt work, locating and destroying invading pathogens.

101

To give you a sense of how important T cells are, keep in mind that the level of T cells is monitored in HIV/AIDS patients to ascertain their state of health.

Foreign substances such as bacteria, viruses, chemicals or pollens are called antigens. Anything that stimulates the body to produce antibodies is an antigen. When T cells come in contact with antigens, they rapidly divide, producing large numbers of new T cells ready to fight that particular antigen.

The B cells work in sync with their cousins the T cells. B cells secured their moniker because they mature in our bone marrow. These are the little guys that produce antibodies, specific proteins that help us recognize and fight infections. Some B cells, called memory cells, survive for years. They have been previously exposed to a specific infection. When that type of infection reoccurs, these memory cells immediately recognize the invader and rouse the appropriate defense system.

Neutrophils, another type of white blood cell, remain our first line of defense against invaders. They defend our bodies by seeking out foreign microorganisms, which they kill and then digest. Although the population of neutrophils doesn't decline with age, their ability to seek and destroy wanes. Chemotherapy, radiation and viral infections can cause their numbers to plunge drastically, resulting in a potentially life-threatening situation called neutropenia. Without enough neutrophils, our bodies have trouble defending against bacterial and fungal infections. A clinical trial conducted in Israel demonstrated that small doses of honey can stave off neutropenia during cancer treatments.[2] (For more information see the chapter on complementing cancer therapy).

Since T cells, B cells and neutrophils keep our immune system running smoothly, we obviously would love to support their efforts. Lab tests demonstrate honey has the potential to increase the numbers of B and T cells in addition to neutrophil counts.[3] A further animal study tested whether honey incorporated into the diet at a rate of 0.8 g per kg of body weight per day significantly increased the production of antibodies when the animals were exposed to two types of invaders: foreign blood and *E. coli*.[4] The production of antibodies, which inactivate antigens by binding to them, increased significantly in response to both invasions.

Rich in antioxidants, honey has great potential to protect the immune system as we age. Researcher Lynne Chepulis decided to test the effects in a long term animal study for her PhD thesis at the University of Waikato in New Zealand.[5] The animals were fed a diet similar in composition to a typical New Zealand diet: 15-16 percent of the total energy in the diet came from protein, 35 percent from fat, and carbohydrates made up the remaining 45-47 percent. The sugar source varied between the three test groups:

1) sugar free diet which incorporated amylose
2) sucrose
3) honeydew honey, a type of honey rich in minerals and antioxidants

After a year on the diet, the animals fed the sucrose or honey diet had significantly higher neutrophil counts than those on the sugar free diet. Most interestingly, the honey fed animals displayed higher levels of lymphocytes, the important white blood cells that help defend our body against disease. The animals fed honey had almost twice as many lymphocytes as the animals on the sugar free diet and 1.3 times more than the sucrose fed group.

Long term consumption of honey seems to thus enhance the immune system's ability to respond to bacterial and fungal infections. Bacterial and fungal infections claim the lives of many elderly, so a functioning immune system is critical as we age.[6] While neutrophil numbers in humans are not believed to decline with age, they do decrease in function over time. Honey could potentially mitigate the waning ability of these important elements of our immune system.

How does honey actually boost our immune system? More research is still needed to definitively answer that question, but one way that honey may boost our immune system is by supporting the establishment of beneficial bifidobacteria in our gut. The antioxidants in honey discussed previously in Chapter 1 may also enhance our immune system.

## STRESS BUSTER

For her PhD research, Lynne Chepulis worked with Dr. Nicola Starkey, an animal behavior psychologist. Together they discovered that a long term honey diet reduced anxiety and improved spatial memory in their animal experiments.

Our health typically deteriorates with increasing age. As each year rolls by our risk of numerous ailments increases: obesity, cardiovascular disease, diabetes and cognitive impairments. All of these disorders have complex roots that involve our genetic make-up, our lifestyle and our environment - no single factor causes any of them. Yet long term changes to our diet have a surprising impact on these serious conditions for better and worse.

Research has shown that prolonged high blood glucose levels cause the body to undergo oxidative stress. Unleashed free radicals damage our precious DNA, proteins and other important cellular components essential to a fully functioning body. Antioxidants work to counter the damage, but as we mature our body is less capable of producing antioxidants.

Free radicals can damage all cells in our body. The brain consumes large amounts of oxygen, which generates higher levels of free radicals, Dr. Starkey explained during her presentation at the First International Symposium on Honey and Human Health, referencing the findings of other researchers.[7] Concentrated free radicals coupled with high levels of polyunsaturated fatty acids in brain cell membranes and low levels of antioxidants leave the brain extremely susceptible to oxidative stress.

Alzheimer patients frequently display increased oxidative damage. Diabetes leaves individuals at a higher risk of dementia and cognitive decline. Even pre-diabetics, who suffer from impaired glucose tolerance, display decreases in working memory, verbal declarative memory and executive functions.

Working memory is the equivalent of a scratch pad. It holds onto and can manipulate vital short term information while we complete a task. We need verbal declarative memory to understand and retain facts and words. Executive function enables us to react and plan; without it we can not adapt to changing situations, anticipate results or plan for the future. Declines in all three leave us failing to comprehend.

While the picture of aging sounds pretty bleak, there is hope for both young and old. People who consume low GI diets show improvement in brain function. Too much glucose in the blood increases the generation of free radicals. When high circulating blood glucose levels occur together with reduced antioxidant production in older individuals, it can lead to cellular brain damage.

Dr. Starkey highlighted research that shows consumption of natural antioxidants may lead to improved mental performance in animals and humans. As discussed previously, honey has been shown to have strong antioxidant properties that are readily available to the human body.[8,9, 10] The animals that received the diet containing honey had significantly lower oxidative damage at the end of the experiment.

## Unforgettable Memory

During the year long trial, the animals were also tested on their ability to remember mazes. The animals consuming honey were much more likely to remember where they had been previously and thus explore new routes than either the sugar or the sugar-free group.

Anxiety and stress increase the generation of free radicals. Using an elevated maze, Starkey and Chepulis tested the level of anxiety their test animals felt. When uneasy, the animals tended to hide in covered sections of the maze; they waltzed out into open sections when relaxed and carefree. The honey fed animals lacked anxiety and accordingly spent much more of their time in open sections and less time in the covered sections than either of the two other groups.

In addition to weight reduction, lower body fat, decreased anxiety, better spatial memory, improved blood sugar levels and reduced oxidative damage (as if that weren't enough!), the honey also led to 15-20 percent higher levels of HDL cholesterol. This is the good type of cholesterol our primary care physicians are keen on elevating. High levels have been linked to reduced risk of coronary heart disease, which affects about 14 million Americans. Plaque, calcium and fatty material build up in our arteries, stopping the flow of blood to the heart. As mentioned in the last chapter, HDL is believed to carry cholesterol away from the arteries back to the liver, where it is passed from the body, reducing the buildup of plaque in our arteries.

While we can't literally turn back the clock, incorporating honey into our diet may potentially help us retain our health for many years, keeping our mind sharp as we age. Obviously more trials confirming the beneficial effects of honey carry over to humans are needed. Unlike drugs that cause serious side effects, honey is a perfectly safe food. In light of the growing body of evidence, we could certainly replace some of our regular sugar consumption with honey.

# *Interlude*

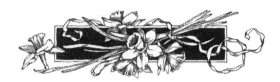

## *Long Live the Queen*

In 1609, Charles Butler, the father of English beekeeping, pays the recently deceased Queen Elizabeth I a lasting tribute by finally putting to rest the falsehood that a king rules a beehive. In his book *The Feminine Monarchie* he correctly states a queen dominates as ruler. In his ground-breaking book, Butler describes the medicinal values of honey:[1]

- For cleansing and disinfecting

- As a laxative and diuretic

- A cough medicine

- An eye balm

- A highly nourishing restorative

- An aphrodisiac

- A preservative

- A mouthwash for ulcers

- A gargle for quinsy (a complication of tonsillitis) and sore throats

- A treatment for snake bites

- A sobering agent for those who have partaken of mild narcotics

- A calming agent after stomach upsets.

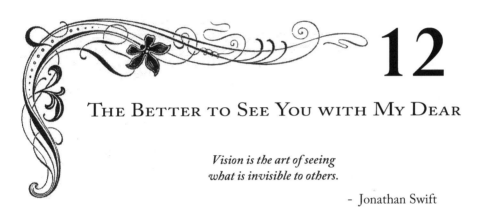

# 12

## THE BETTER TO SEE YOU WITH MY DEAR

*Vision is the art of seeing
what is invisible to others.*

- Jonathan Swift

*V*ision must be our most precious sense. Sight lets us experience our environment in a dazzling array of colors and shapes. Our eyes enable us to enjoy the swirls of magenta that melt into apricot and mauve when the setting sun sets the sky aflame. We instantly recognize a loved one moving through a crowd because of slight nuances in movement.

Our visual acuity fades with time. Many of us require glasses to help us continue to see clearly. Since antiquity doctors have used honey to treat disorders of the eye, including infections and cataracts. The Babylonians and Assyrians applied prescriptions containing honey to heal eye troubles.

Around 250 BC, Zenon worked as an employee of Apollonios, an important advisor to Ptolemy II in charge of the treasury. Zenon travelled extensively, frequently taking honey on his voyages. In a letter he received from Dromon, the latter reports:

> *according to Zenon's instructions he is taking good care that his employees are not molested. Before Zenon sails up the river in good health, let him order one of his people to buy a kotyle (about 9 gallons) of Attic honey; for Dromon has been commanded by the god to use this as a medicament for his eyes.*

Beekeepers still harvest the famous medicinal honey when the wild thyme bursts into bloom on the rocky mountainsides of Greece, once part of Attica. Aristotle discussed the benefits of honey in his book *Historia Animalium*, also known as *On the History of Animals*:

> *When thyme blooms, and the cells are filled with honey, it does not thicken. The gold colored honey is nice, but the white one is not purely from thyme, yet it is good for the eyes and ulcers.*[1]

The *Leechbook of Bald*, one of the most detailed glimpses into Saxon herbal remedies from approximately 900 AD, recommends honey as a constituent of an eye salve. More recently an article published in India in 1945, calls honey that bees make from lotus blossoms a "panacea"; a universal cure-all for eye diseases.[2] An Indian eye surgeon at Rangaraya Medical College, India has found that to be true and successfully treated bacterial ulcers of the cornea with honey.[3]

The Bambara of Mali frequently live in large dwellings with up to 60 extended family members. When someone comes down with measles they traditionally apply honey to the eyes to protect the cornea form scarring.[4] Perhaps if more knew of this folk remedy measles would not be one of the leading causes of visual impairment and blindness in children of Africa.[5]

## A HORSE, OF COURSE

While the examples above clearly demonstrate the historical use of honey on human eyes, the application was never limited to two legged creatures. Honey saved a number of horses from blindness. Vigerius reports:

> *I have cured a Horse stone blind with Honey and Salt and a little crock of a pot mixed. In less than three daies (days), it hath eaten off a tough filme, and the Horse never complained after.*[6]

A beekeeper confirms the effectiveness of treating a horse with honey by sharing the following experience in a 1937 issue of *American Bee Journal*:

> *I had a horse going blind with a white film over his eye which seemed to hurt. His eye was shut and watered. I dipped white honey into his eye with a feather for several nights. In a day or so the film was gone and the eye looked bright and good.*[7]

## SOUTH OF THE BORDER

In South America, many harvest honey from stingless bees. Numerous South American cultures believe honey from stingless bees cures eye disorders.[8] This honey has a much higher water content and different properties including greater acidity than honey from *Apis mellifera*, the European honey bee kept by beekeepers in the United States.

Honey from stingless bees, called *Meliponini*, is frequently used to treat cataracts. This ancient tradition dates back to the Mayans, who recorded the medical use of honey in their pharmacopeia. Throughout the world, over 93 million people have limited sight due to cataracts, which cause a clouding of the lens.[9] Thirty-nine million people are blind in the world[10] and half lost their sight due to cataracts.[11]

Cataracts usually start out small, causing little impact on our vision. A build-up of proteins on the lens of the eye stops it from focusing light sharply. Our vision becomes blurred, like peering through smeared glass and the world starts to resemble an impressionist painting with no definitive lines. One of the first signs people tend to notice is that lights at night have more glare.

When cataracts start impairing vision, doctors will often recommend the lens be removed surgically. Complications can arise after the operation as the outermost layer of cells clump on the capsule that contained your lens.

If you could delay the onset of cataracts by 10 years, you would reduce the number of necessary cataract operations by 45 percent.[12] The lens tries to protect itself from cataracts via antioxidants and maintaining equal salt and water levels on the inside and outside of the eye.[13]

Applying eye treatments can help delay the onset of cataracts. Meliponini honey contains a wide array of flavonoids. While flavonoids are best known for their antioxidant properties, they also influence human health in other ways. They can inhibit enzymes involved in the clouding of eyes, stopping them short and thus halting the formation of cataracts.

A number of stingless bee honey flavonoids act as anticataract agents, inhibiting enzymes involved in cataract development.[14] Both laboratory and animal experiments have confirmed stingless bee honey flavonoids have properties that minimize cataract formation.[15]

The ancient Mayans might have enjoyed learning that stingless bee honey from Venezuela often contains the flavonoid luteolin. In lab tests this specific type of flavonoid and its derivatives stopped the formation of cataracts.[16] Because of the widespread use of honey for eye disorders in South America, a large variety of stingless bee honey eye drops are available for sale. Stingless bee eye drops could be applied before surgical intervention to reduce cataract size.

## RUSSIAN RESEARCH

Before the fall of the U.S.S.R., many Russian scientists investigated the properties of various products from the hive, including honey. They published numerous papers on their work with honey as an eye salve.[17] Honey proved especially effective against treating various lesions and ulcerations of the cornea.

In a clinical trial completed in the early 1990s, Russian doctors treated developing cataracts in seniors with pure honey diluted in water for three months. This was done once or twice annually.[18] Throughout the year, the eyes were treated with vitamin drops. One hundred and eight patients were monitored for two to 15 years. Over 95.5 percent treated retained at least minimal vision of 20/200. In 55.9 percent the vision did not continue to deteriorate during future follow-ups, while vision was preserved in only 35.3 percent of the controls.

## ISLAMIC MEDICINE

Many Muslims, who follow the teachings of the Koran and the Holy Hadith, believe in the curative properties of honey:

> And thy Lord taught the bee to build its cells in hills, on trees and in (men's) habitations ... there issues from within their bodies a drink of varying colors, wherein is healing for mankind. Verily in this is a Sign for those who give thought.

The prophet Mohammed is quoted as saying:

> Honey is a remedy for every illness and the Koran is a remedy for

*all illness of the mind, therefore I recommend to you both remedies, the Koran and honey.*

Since honey carries such high regard amongst Muslims, it should be no surprise that doctors implement honey for medical purposes. A scientific study reported in the Bulletin of Islamic Medicine in 1982 reported positive results with 102 patients who had not responded to conventional treatments for a range of eye disorders.[19] The patients suffered from inflammation of the cornea (keratitis), pink eye, an inflammation of the outermost layer of the eye and the inner surface of the eyelid (conjunctivitis), and inflammation of the eyelids (blepharitis). All were treated with honey applied to the lower eyelid.

The simple honey treatment caused improvement in 85 percent, while the other 15 percent showed no sign of deterioration. The only drawback: some patients experienced a short stinging sensation and slight redness of the eye shortly after application. The pain must have been negligible, as neither side effect caused any of the patients to stop the treatments.

## ALLEVIATING DRY EYES

A recent clinical trial conducted in Australia used honey to treat individuals suffering from dry eyes.[20] This disorder can be caused by tear deficiency or by a disease of the small meibomian gland in the eyelid that makes an oily lubricant. The eyes were treated three times daily with a topical application of antibacterial honey.

At the start of the study, researchers isolated bacteria from the corner of the patient's eyes. Those suffering from dry eye had significantly higher bacterial counts than healthy subjects. The honey treatments reduced the bacterial load so that by the end of three months the number of bacteria isolated from the 66 dry eye patients did not vary from those of the 18 healthy individuals. The researchers concluded that honey deserves more attention and further studies for its ability to help heal chronic eye surface diseases.

## FUTURE DIRECTIONS

Much folk medicine and anecdotal evidence highlights the potential benefits of using honey to treat eye disorders. More modern research and larger clinical trials should be conducted to clearly delineate in what conditions honey may help, as the first trials certainly look promising.

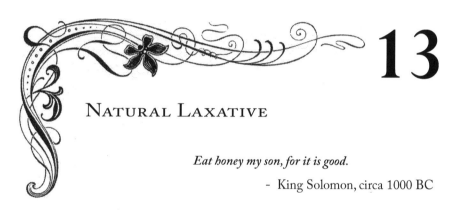

# 13

## NATURAL LAXATIVE

*Eat honey my son, for it is good.*

- King Solomon, circa 1000 BC

*C*onstipation has plagued humans for centuries. Maimonides—physician to the demanding sultan of Egypt, his large harem and countless children—was kept quite busy maintaining the health of his employer and abnormally numerous family in the 12th century. Forced to flee his home in Spain as a child when the zealous Muslim Almohades dynasty came to power, Maimonides and his family fled to Morocco, then Israel, before finally settling in Egypt. His brother, a jewelry merchant, perished on a voyage across the Indian Ocean, taking the family fortune down into his watery grave.

Obliged to stop his religious studies to earn a living, Maimonides learned the medical profession. Despite his hardships, he never lost his religious faith. A highly admired Jewish rabbi, he authored many texts including the *Guide to the Perplexed*, in which he attempted to reconcile scientific knowledge with his religious beliefs. Despite his long hours at the sultan's palace and his dedication to the faithful who sought his advice on the Sabbath, he came up with a solution to constipation over 800 years ago.

> *How can a person heal his intestines if they are slightly consti-pated? …If he is an old man, he should drink honey mixed with warm water in the morning and wait approximately four hours, and then he should eat his meal. He should do this for one day or three or four days if it is necessary, until his intestines soften* (and move freely).[1]

A common folk remedy for constipation in many cultures, honey works as a mild laxative. In Karachi, Pakistan mothers often feed new-borns honey as they believe it reduces colic and acts as a laxative.[2]

Due to widespread use of this natural laxative solution in Greece, researchers decided to see if there was any substance to the myth. In their study, 20 healthy individuals volunteered to put the folk medicine to the test. The researchers concluded, "Honey may have a laxative effect on nor-mal subjects because of incomplete fructose absorption." The body does not digest some of the fructose content of the honey, so it passes through the gastrointestinal tract, lubricating the system.

While it seems contrary to logic that one product can combat oppos-ing ailments, honey has effectively treated both constipation and diarrhea since antiquity. One of the greatest Roman medical writers, Aulus Cor-nelius Celsus, penned an encyclopedic reference in approximately 25 BC. Only his treatise on medicine *De medicina* survives, which provides a fascinating glimpse into the medical practices of Alexandria.

Celsus took a pragmatic view to experimenting on human subjects, believing society should sacrifice a few criminals for the health of the greater populous. "Nor is it, as most people say, cruel that in the execu-tion of criminals, and but a few of them, we should seek remedies for innocent people of all future ages."[3] According to him the "bowels are moved by uncooked honey".[4] While Celsus couldn't have known incom-plete fructose absorption caused the bowels to move, he did recognize honey's laxative effect.

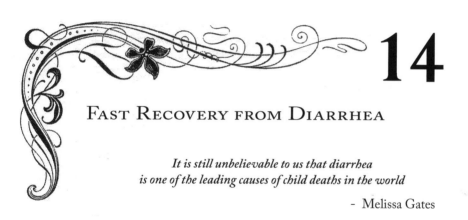

# 14

## FAST RECOVERY FROM DIARRHEA

*It is still unbelievable to us that diarrhea*
*is one of the leading causes of child deaths in the world*

- Melissa Gates

*T*he Roman medical writer Aulus Cornelius Celsus, introduced in the previous chapter, also mentioned honey as a remedy for diarrhea, explaining how "the bowels are confined by cooked honey".[1] The tradition of healing the embarrassing and often incapacitating condition with honey continues to this day in the Islamic world. Many Muslims abide by recommendations in the Hadith, the oral records transcribed after the prophet's death. "The Holy Hadith records the Muslim prophet Mohammed instructing a man afflicted with diarrhea to take honey."[2]

Infectious diarrhea inflicted our ancestors long before we had a written language. As cultivation of arable land developed and we settled into communal housing, we unintentionally became viable hosts and carriers of diarrhea causing microorganisms.[3]

If the cause of diarrhea stems from a bacterial infection, ingesting honey can be very effective in shortening the duration of the uncomfortable and sometimes downright painful affliction. One medical study involved 169 infants and children admitted into the hospital for gastroenteritis, the medical term used to describe an inflammation of the stomach lining and the intestines. [4] Typical symptoms include nausea, vomiting, diarrhea, and cramps. Some of the patients received a rehydration solution that contained five percent honey, while others were administered a standard glucose solution.

Diarrhea caused by bacteria persisted for only 58 hours in the honey group, compared to 93 hours for those treated with the standard glucose solution. Honey shortened the duration of illness from almost four days down to just under two-and-a-half. When the children suffered from a viral infection, the honey solution produced identical effects as standard glucose solution, suggesting the alleviation in the bacterial cases was due to honey's antibacterial properties.[5, 6, 7]

The World Health Organization estimates diarrhea kills 1.8 million people per year. Ninety percent of those who die are children that have not yet celebrated their fifth birthday.[8] Children are highly susceptible because their small body size and high energy needs hasten dehydration.

Doctors normally treat diarrhea through simple rehydration. The World Health Organization recommends using a salt and glucose solution to restore the body.[9] As seen in the clinical trial described above, a five percent honey solution proved just as effective in rehydrating patients as the glucose-salt formula.[10] The additional fructose content in honey promotes water uptake and minimizes sodium uptake, avoiding the risk of too much salt circulating in the blood stream. While glucose causes the body to lose potassium, fructose promotes uptake of this important mineral.[11]

## Montezuma's Revenge

Citizens of developing countries most frequently suffer from watery bowel movements. Yet globalization, the ease of travel and the rapid movement of people has led to increased occurrences of traveler's diarrhea. Also known as Montezuma's revenge, bacterial diarrhea strikes down individuals when they come in contact with previously unencountered pathogens.

While locals have developed immunity to the bacteria through regular contact, a foreigner's system has yet to be hardened.

Honey reins in the nasty effects of Montezuma's revenge. But how does it work? As explained above, honey promotes sodium and water absorption through its high sugar content.[12] By encouraging water absorption, honey may in effect be dehydrating diarrhea into normal stool, helping to alleviate the issue. Honey also stamps out common bacteria that cause bouts of diarrhea, including numerous strains of E. coli, salmonella and shigella.[13]

Research on treating horses afflicted by diarrhea with honey suggests, "The effectiveness of honey in treating diarrhea may be due to it effecting repair of the intestinal mucosa (the linings of the intestines) damaged by the infection."[14] According to honey researcher Dr. Peter Molan from New Zealand, honey's anti-inflammatory properties soothe the inflamed tissue, helping to restore the delicate lining of the intestine.[15]

## Honey And Yogurt

While honey has proven especially effective against bacterial diarrhea, fermented milk products rich in probiotics such as yogurt help against other types of diarrhea.[16] "Since the early 20th century, it has been hypothesized that live bacterial cultures, such as those used for the fermentation of dairy products, may offer benefits in preventing and treating diarrhea."[17]

With over 180 substances, including amino acids, vitamins, minerals and enzymes, honey satisfies the complex nutritional needs of the lactic acid bacteria in yogurt.[18] Most honey also has an abundance of fructose in relationship to glucose. This excess fructose passes on through the gut, where the simple sugar provides food to the beneficial bacteria that colonize our approximately 30 foot long gastrointestinal tract. These properties make honey a fabulous prebiotic that supports the growth and longevity of the lactic acid bacteria [19] both in yogurt and in our intestinal tract. Probiotics prove useful in the prevention and treatment of diarrhea.[20] Both pre and probiotics are discussed in greater detail in chapter 9, Feeding the Flora.

According to Kathene Johnson-Henry, research project manager of Gastroenterology for the Hospital of Sick Children in Toronto, Canada; "Honey may have the advantage of a dual purpose: it a) decreases the total number of pathogens in the gut and b) increases the number of beneficial bacteria in the commensal flora (the microorganisms of the gut). This could prove beneficial in some gastrointestinal disorders (such as traveler's diarrhea)."[21]

To prevent Montezuma's revenge, folk remedies prescribe both honey and yogurt. Perhaps our ancestors recognized the benefits of combining yogurt and honey, as many traditional recipes mix these two ingredients. The dessert menu in most authentic Greek restaurants serves up a tantalizing treat of thick, rich slightly tangy yogurt drizzled with sweet, luscious honey. You might want to keep some on hand for the next time you face a questionable meal.

# *Interlude*

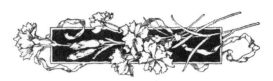

## *Ambrosia and Vegetarianism*

The Greeks considered honey to be the food of their mighty gods. Their gods also drank ambrosia, a fermented honey beverage commonly known as mead and most likely the earliest alcoholic beverage. The preferred food of their gods played a substantial role in Greek medicine.

Hippocrates recommended honey for lowering fever and for cooling the blood. His students knew over 300 honey recipes, 60 of which were drinks such as sour-honey; a mixture of vinegar and honey:[1]

> *The drink to be employed should there be any pain is oxymel (vinegar and honey). If there be great thirst, give hydromel (water and honey).*[2]

During the Olympic Games in Ancient Greece, the exhausted male athletes replenished their energy by drinking water mixed with honey. Composed predominantly of the simple sugars glucose and fructose, honey delivers a two-fold punch of energy: the body uses glucose immediately, while fructose must first be converted to glucose, thus acting as a slow release energy form.

Perhaps honey helped stimulate the mind of the great mathematician and philosopher Pythagoras. He and his disciples were vegetarians. The word Pythagorean described people who abstained from meat, until the first vegetarian society coined the word "vegetarian" in the 1840s. When asked the secret of his great age, Pythagoras credited it to his regular use of honey:

> *Bread and honey was the chief foods of the Pythagoreans according to the statement of Aristoxenes (c. 350 BC) who says that those who eat this for breakfast were free from disease all of the lives.*[3]

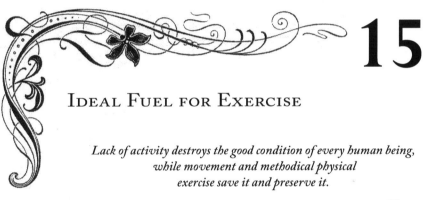

# 15

## IDEAL FUEL FOR EXERCISE

*Lack of activity destroys the good condition of every human being,
while movement and methodical physical
exercise save it and preserve it.*

- Plato

*H*eaded for the track and want a refreshing thirst quencher? Why not follow in the footsteps of the original Olympic athletes, who replenished their energy by drinking honey water?[1] Instead of pouring your money into expensive sports drinks, add a spoonful of honey into your water bottle. Composed of two simple sugars, glucose and fructose, honey provides the body with instant energy plus a slow burning reserve. The body uses glucose immediately, while it must first convert fructose to glucose, releasing energy slowly. For the body to use regular sugar, composed entirely of sucrose, it must break the complex sugar into simple sugars, depleting the body's own energy stores.

Many athletes have discovered this double-packed-punch of honey, relying on it to fuel their bodies before, during and after endurance sports. "Honey's unique carbohydrate composition (approximately equal amounts of fructose and glucose) may render it the perfect pre-exercise food. Research published in the Journal of Applied Physiology suggests that carbohydrates that are lower on the glycemic index (GI) may reduce the incidence of rebound hypoglycemia and provide sustained carbohydrate availability during exercise."[2]

By eating carbohydrates before and during exercise, you prevent fatigue hitting you too soon. Consuming carbohydrates after exercise helps to replenish lost stores of glycogen, so that the body can continue to supply the brain and muscles with energy.

Honey provides 17 grams of carbohydrate per tablespoon, making it an excellent fuel source. In an expedition to Siberia, a group of fur traders schlepped along 2.5 tons of honey according to a record from 1497.[3] The honey served as a concentrated energy food source, helping the group survive the extreme climatic conditions in Siberia.

While most of us aren't planning on trekking through Siberia, a shot of honey in water makes for an excellent sports drink for the casual sport enthusiast. If you prefer lemon or limeade, squirt in half a fresh lemon or lime as well.

Have you ever looked at the nutrition label of a sports drink? The ingredients of Gatorade Raspberry Lemonade are water, sucrose syrup, glucose-fructose syrup, citric acid, natural and artificial flavors, salt, sodium citrate, monopotassium phosphate, ester gum, sucrose acetate isobutyrate, red 40 and blue 1. Food labels always list ingredients in quantitative order, starting with the primary ingredient.

Along with water, you are gulping mainly sucrose syrup, which is plain white sugar dissolved in water. Some glucose-fructose syrup tossed in gives the benefits of the simple sugars in honey, without the added vitamins, minerals and antioxidants this natural sweetener provides. To make up for the lack of minerals, producers of the well-known thirst quenchers throw in some salt and potassium, both of which occur naturally in honey. Citric acid gives the water slight acidity to enhance fluid uptake. Again, this occurs naturally with honey, which ranges in acidity value from a pH of 3.2 to 4.5.[4]

Those artificial food colors do make the beverage look attractive, but if you are thirsty and don't have a sports drink lying around, why not whip up your own with some honey?

## CITRUS THIRST QUENCHER

### Ingredients
1/2 cup honey
1/4 cup fresh squeezed lemon or lime juice
7 and 1/2 cups water

### Directions
Mix ingredients in a large pitcher. Slightly warm water will help dissolve the honey. Then chill if desired.

## ENDURANCE SPORTS

According to sports nutritionist Stuart McInnes and his chemist father Mike McInnes, the key to success for endurance athletes lies in properly preparing your body for exercise beforehand. When the heart pumps at an accelerated rate, the body needs access to glucose. It pulls glucose stores from the liver. Should you try to refuel the body using sugary sports drinks and high glycemic carbohydrates, "some 60-70 grams of glucose will be absorbed rapidly and blood sugar will rocket upwards. This is dangerous and a tidal wave of insulin will be released to deal with this."[5]

When an athlete resumes activity after a short break of fifteen minutes, blood sugar levels plummet. Having already depleted the liver stores, instead of pulling additional glucose from fat stores, the body steals proteins from muscles. So if you are exercising to lose weight, or to bulk up muscles, you must keep your liver fueled. Honey, fresh fruits and vegetables provide the perfect ratio of glucose and fructose.

A clinical trial tested nine male endurance athletes to see how well they performed in three simulated 64 km timed cycling trials.[6] Consuming honey helped them shave minutes off their racing time compared to a placebo. In high profile races where even seconds count, honey improved the cyclists' times by approximately 2 ½ minutes. The researchers concluded that a honey gel may prove to be an effective energy source for endurance athletes.

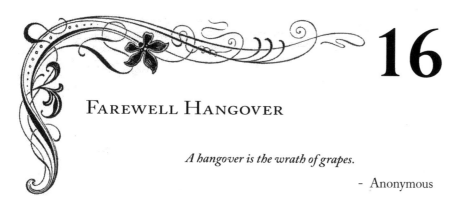

# 16

## FAREWELL HANGOVER

*A hangover is the wrath of grapes.*

- Anonymous

Drink too much on an empty stomach? After a night on the town, does the bright morning light make you feel like you want to bury your head back under the covers? Ease yourself out of the pain by spreading a thick layer of honey on a piece of toast. A press release published by the Royal Society of Chemistry in England found that eating honey on toast helps speed up recovery from alcoholic over-indulgence the night before.

The chemistry of the remedy undoes the mischief alcohol creates in our bodies. Our bodies convert alcohol into the toxic chemical acetalde-hyde, which results in a vicious headache and can bring on nausea. The hangover dampens our mood and makes us extra sensitive to noise until our system has converted the poison into less harmful chemicals.

According to Dr. John Emsley of the Royal Society of Chemistry, "The happiness comes from alcohol; the hangover comes from acetaldehyde. This is the toxic chemical into which alcohol is converted by the body and it causes a throbbing headache, nausea, and maybe even vomiting. The hangover disappears as the acetaldehyde is slowly converted to less toxic chemicals. That's the science."[1]

While most Americans have overindulged on alcohol at least once in their lifetime, they may not be aware how expensive a hangover can be. When hangover pain overwhelms, many Americans call in sick or perform poorly at the office. The unexpected absenteeism and poor job performance costs $148 billion annually, an average of $2,000 per worker.[2]

Honey left out in an open vessel draws in moisture and ferments, and so created our ancestor's first alcoholic beverage in the form of mead. Prehistoric people probably first faced a hangover soon after accidentally discovering the pleasures of alcohol. Famed writers of ancient Egypt and Greece recorded descriptions of hangovers, as did the Old Testament.[3]

The British writer William Hickey described the aftereffects of overindulgence most vividly in 1768:

> My first return of sense or recollection was upon waking in a strange, dismal-looking room, my head aching horridly, pains of a violent nature in every limb, and deadly sickness at the stomach. From the latter I was in some degree relieved by a very copious vomiting. Getting out of bed, I looked out of the window in the room, but saw nothing but the backs of old houses, from which various miserable emblems of poverty were displayed. …At that moment I do not believe in the world there existed a more wretched creature than myself.[4]

Typically a hangover erupts when the alcohol level in our blood starts to wane. As a result we feel exhausted and experience increased sensitivity to light and sound. Our head pounds, our eyes are bloodshot, our muscles ache and we crave something to drink to cool our parched throats. Depending on the severity, we may experience elevated blood pressure, rapid heartbeats, tremors and sweating. The room tends to spin. Depression and anxiety can take root. The slightest intrusion into our space makes us irritable. The peak of our discomfort levels out when our blood alcohol concentration finally returns to zero, although hangover symptoms can continue for an additional 24 hours.[5]

It seems fitting that honey, which fermented into the world's first alcoholic beverage, also provides the body with the nutrients we so desperately need to recover after alcoholic overindulgence. Fructose, abundant in most honeys, has been shown to reduce the length of time it takes alcohol to leave the blood, potentially shrinking the length of a hangover.[6] "The fructose of honey competes with the alcohol for receptor sites during metabolism," according to Dr. Merle Diamond of the Diamond Headache Clinic in Chicago. She has been a headache specialist for twenty years.[7] "Honey helps the body metabolize the alcohol more slowly. This avoids the abrupt change in alcohol levels that triggers the headache of a hangover."[8]

In addition to messing with our metabolism, alcohol also irritates the stomach lining. Honey contains potent anti-inflammatory properties that can help soothe away upper abdominal pain and nausea.[9]

When binge drinking people often forget to eat. Alcohol consumption alters the smooth functioning of our internal system, especially the liver, and low glucose levels are often the result. Since glucose is the primary energy source for the brain, starving the brain can contribute to hangover symptoms like fatigue, weakness and mood swings.[10] Luckily the other predominant sugar in honey is glucose, which provides the body with instant energy.

So before you head out for a long night on the town with your drinking buddies, you may want to stock up on a jar of honey. "Here's my headache cocktail, no pun intended," Dr. Diamond said with a hearty laugh. While her remedy works, she was quick to first point out that she doesn't recommend alcoholic overindulgence. "Eat some honey on crackers before you go out. Then stick to white wine, gin or vodka. While drinking, also consume fruit juice. When you come home, eat some more honey on crackers, take two Aleves and you won't wake up with a headache. It really works."[11]

Other tips to help to avoid a hangover: Start your night on the town with a glass of milk. The milk slows down the absorption of alcohol, so less acetaldehyde builds up in the body at any given time.[12]

Avoid dark liquors and order white wine, vodka or gin instead. These contain very few congeners; compounds that add an extra whammy to a hangover. Red wine, brandy and whiskey contain both ethanol and methanol. Methanol lingers in the body, as ethanol inhibits the body from breaking it down. When the body does finally break down methanol, it first creates formaldehyde—that noxious smelling fluid used to preserve organs—and then formic acid, both of which are toxic to humans in high concentrations.[13]

Consume a few non-alcoholic beverages during your night on the town. Alcohol is a diuretic, causing frequent visits to the restroom. For every four alcoholic drinks you consume, you void about a quart of water. The alcohol stops your body from producing a hormone that regulates urination. A few extra glasses of juice or water will help rehydrate you. Be sure to drink at least a pint of water before you doze off to sleep, as dehydration increases the intensity of a hangover.[14,15] If you like, swirl in a large spoonful of honey to replenish lost glucose and fructose. You should wake up symptom free in the morning.

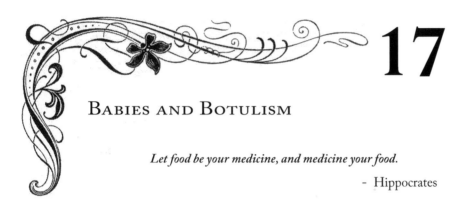

# 17

## BABIES AND BOTULISM

*Let food be your medicine, and medicine your food.*

- Hippocrates

$\mathcal{S}$pores pervade our world. One of these, *Clostridium botulinum*, can cause infant botulism when provided with an anaerobic environment (lacking air or oxygen) in which to proliferate. Ubiquitous in soil, air, dust and raw agricultural products, *C. botulinum* spores occasionally end up in honey.

Designed to survive inhospitable conditions, spores instigate no damage in this asexual reproductive form. The acidic environment of the digestive tract in children above the age of one and in adults prevents botulism spores from germinating.

But in young children, whose gut lacks intestinal flora, *C. botulinum* spores may germinate and colonize the large intestine, producing the toxin botulin that blocks nerve function. Often the first sign of botulism in an infant is constipation. Since the toxin blocks the transmission of nerve impulses, other symptoms include general weakness, waning sucking, crying and swallowing ability, difficulty breathing and eventual paralysis. If treated appropriately, a child can make a full recover.

A rare disease, infant botulism affects few children. Since 1973, "71 cases of infant botulism have been reported annually to the US Centers for Disease Control and Prevention."[1] The chances of a baby contracting this illness are less than one in 12,000.[2]

As stated above, C. botulinum spores pervade our environment. Dust remains the most common source of contamination. Doctors recommend parents not feed honey and corn syrup to infants before their first birthday, because these are *avoidable* sources of possible spores.

In contradiction, many cultural traditions feed honey to newborn infants as their first food. "From the beginning of recorded history, and probably earlier, honey has been given to newborn children as part of the birth rite in many regions of the world."[3] Greeks, Indians, Germans, and Hebrews engaged in this common practice:[4]

> *The newborn child was regarded as a "soul" or "spirit" until it had received food; if a child's mouth had once been smeared with honey, it might not be killed. …In early Christian times it was used immediately after baptism.*[5]

The custom of feeding honey to infants persists in many countries to this day. In Egypt, a survey conducted between 1998 and 2002 found that "545 out of 719 mothers (75.8 percent) gave bee honey orally to their 1,525 infants at least once before the age of one year without mortality or significant morbidity that could be attributed to botulism."[6]

Honey has long been associated with good health and strength. "In India and many other parts of the world honey is given to newborn babies during the first few days of life as a special tonic, particularly if they were born weak or prematurely."[7]

Because C. botulinum spores have on occasion been detected in honey, most commercially sold honey states that it should not be fed to children under one-year of age. Unfortunately many people mistakenly believe that since honey is not recommended for young children, it cannot be beneficial for anyone. This false assumption maligns honey's good name.

Many European countries refuse to print a warning on honey labels, as any raw agricultural product, including honey, can contain the botulism causing spores. They feel singling out honey is unfair. In stark contrast to the United States, Europeans still commonly feed honey to infants as numerous medicinal benefits have been linked to this ancient custom.

Clinical studies completed throughout the 20th century noted numerous benefits for infants when honey was added to their diet. The infants absorbed honey faster than sugar, yet their blood sugar levels returned to normal sooner. Honey also aided in the absorption of calcium and magnesium from milk.[8]

The addition of honey to milk raised hemoglobin levels in infants.[9] Hemoglobins are shuttle proteins attached to your red blood cells that permit oxygen to be transported from the lungs throughout the body. Low levels are associated with fatigue and weariness.

The number of intestinal flora, the good bacteria, improved with honey consumption. Premature babies did surprisingly well when fed honey, improving in weight gain and development.[10,11] The addition of honey to the infant diet, instead of sucrose, resulted in reduced vomiting[12] and fewer incidences of diarrhea.[13] Some infant formulas also contained honey instead of corn syrup for many years, a practice that stopped in the 1970s.

A study completed in the 21st century in Italy found that honey significantly reduced infant crying.[14] In the past it was common practice to dip a child's pacifier in honey. But since pacifiers frequently attract dust, this habit fell out of favor with growing fears of infant botulism.

Most infant botulism can be traced back to the ingestion of dust. A key study conducted in Pennsylvania "identified breast-feeding as the major link with the disease. Honey was determined to not be a causative factor, with environmental conditions (soil, dust) implicated as the major and unavoidable source of spores."[15]

According to research done in New Zealand,[16] gamma-irradiated honey contains no botulism spores. So if you wish to feed your child spore-free honey, look for gamma irradiated honey. Nursing mothers may too benefit from the use of honey. Covering the cracked sore nipples of nursing mothers with honey soaked bandages prevented them from becoming infected.[17]

By the time you celebrate your child's first birthday, you can let your child feast on nature's first sweetener. Your child will have developed normal microflora in his or her gut, making honey a perfectly safe food.

# *Interlude*

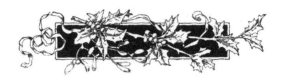

## *Eros and his Arrows of Love*

The Greek god Eros, known to the Romans as Cupid, possesses the power to shoot arrows of love into the hearts of men and gods. Does the mischievous spreader of passion dip his sweet arrows of love in honey? According to some legends, the tip receives a kiss of honey to sweeten its sting.

Honey and Eros appear in a verse attributed to Plato:

> *He [Eros] lay among the rose blooms smiling, bound fast by sleep, and above him the tawny bees were sprinkling on his dainty lips honey dripping from the comb.[1]*

The God of Love adored this golden sweetness and went to great lengths to obtain a taste. Theocritus tells the tale of Eros stealing honey from a hive in his Idyll XIX:

*Love Stealing Honey:*

> *Once thievish Love the honeyed hives would rob,*
> *When a bee stung him: soon he felt a throb*
> *Through all his finger-tips, and, wild with pain,*
> *Blew on his hands and stamped and jumped in vain.*
> *To Aphrodite then he told his woe:*
> *'How can a thing so tiny hurt one so?'*
> *She smiled and said; 'Why thou'rt a tiny thing,*
> *As is the bee; yet sorely thou canst sting.'[2]*

Aphrodite, who the Romans called Venus, was the mother of Eros. When he runs to her for comfort after being stung, she scolds the boy with a smile for his mischievousness. To her the pain the bees inflict is similar to the pain of her son's darts. This legend irrevocably links sweetness and honey with love and the hint of pain. The words of Theocritus inspired myriad artists including Dürer and Cranach the Elder. Picasso later reworked Cranach's theme, depicting the identical pose of Venus and Love in his own style.

Numerous poets retold the myth of *Cupid the Honey Thief*, including the Irish poet Thomas Moore in his *Ode XXXV, Cupid Once Upon a Bed*. Moore was a friend and contemporary of Lord Byron, the Irish poet, and became steward of his famous friend's memoirs. Moore sold Byron's work to the publisher Murray for £2,100, who agreed to honor Bryon's wish and only publish them posthumously. When Byron passed, his family begged Murray and Moore not to publish the candid autobiographical work. Accordingly, Murray burned the Byron memoir and the honorable Moore repaid the publisher the considerable sum of £2,100.

A beloved favorite of the gentry, invited to amuse the lords and ladies with his verse and songs, Moore may have been quite well equipped to write on the topic of love:

> *Cupid once upon a bed*
> *Of roses laid his weary head;*
> *Luckless urchin not to see*
> *Within the leaves a slumbering bee;*
> *The bee awaked--with anger wild*
> *The bee awaked, and stung the child.*
> *Loud and piteous are his cries;*
> *To Venus quick he runs, he flies;*
> *"Oh mother!--I am wounded through--*
> *I die with pain--in sooth I do!*
> *Stung by some little angry thing,*
> *Some serpent on a tiny wing--*
> *A bee it was--for once, I know,*
> *I heard a rustic call it so."*
> *Thus he spoke, and she the while,*
> *Heard him with a soothing smile;*

*Then said, "My infant, if so much*
*Thou feel the little wild-bee's touch,*
*How must the heart, ah, Cupid be,*
*The hapless heart that's stung by thee!"*

One might conclude a honey bee sting is only as painful as the kiss of love, yet many people have an irrational fear of honey bees, born from a sting long ago. Unfortunately, wasps dole out stings that are wrongly attributed to honey bees, besmirching their good name.

As no honey bees originally existed in North America, the colonists imported the European honey bee to pollinate their crops. The European honey bee still kept by beekeepers today, will only sting to defend her colony or when battling for her life. A sting is a death sentence to a honey bee, as her barbed stinger stays behind in our flesh. A modified ovipositor, the stinger was once an egg-laying organ that through the course of history evolved to eject venom instead of eggs. The stinger and the attached muscles continue to pump venom, even after the honey bee struggles away to die.

Should you ever be stung by a honey bee, you will find the stinger left behind in your skin. Don't follow the natural impulse to pick it out! The bulbous projection at the top contains a venom sack. By squeezing it with your fingers, you inject the venom into your body in the same manner as a syringe. Instead, remove a stinger by flicking the barb out using your fingernail or the edge of a credit card.

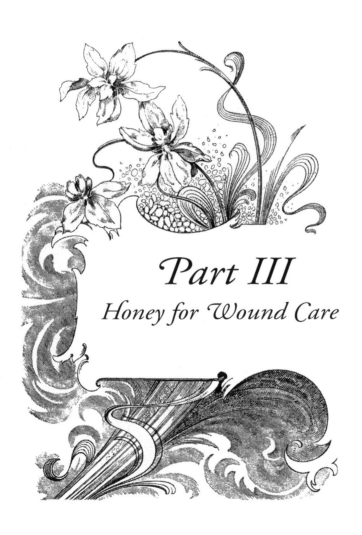

# Part III
## *Honey for Wound Care*

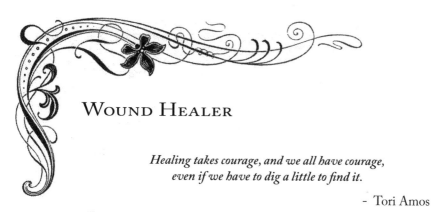

# WOUND HEALER

*Healing takes courage, and we all have courage,*
*even if we have to dig a little to find it.*

- Tori Amos

*T*he nurse hands the newborn girl, swaddled in soft cloth and screaming with all the vivacity her little lungs can muster, into her mother's outstretched arms. The tiny child struggles inside the covers, shocked by the sudden bright light after the warmth and darkness of the womb. The mother leans forward and kisses the small fist clenched tight, the hand that she watched grow and take shape in the ultrasounds during her pregnancy.

For most mothers the pain of giving birth slips from the mind as they hold their infant for the first time, knowing they will soon be headed home. But for Melanie, the struggle had just begun[1] for her daughter Katarina had been born with a malformed spinal canal that protruded from her back and required surgery. Doctors carefully removed the projecting tissues, leaving an open wound. Melanie—unable to help—watched her daughter sleeping on her stomach in the intensive care unit. The wound stagnated and developed three different types of resistant bacteria. *Klebsiella oxytoca,* a common culprit of wound infections in neonatal intensive care units, took up residence and transformed Katarina's back into a battleground.

To beat back the infection, doctors hooked up IVs, piping an antibiotic into the newborn. When that drug failed, they tried another in combination with conventional wound care treatments. But the multiresistant bacteria refused to die, leaving Katarina's back a raw, open wound.

Days slowly trickled into weeks, weeks into months without any signs of improvement. Three months passed and Katarina's back made no progress. Frustrated and desperate to help her child, Melanie read all she could about wound care. She discovered that Dr. Arne Simon, a pediatric oncologist, applied medical grade honey to heal the wounds of his young, cancer patients. To Melanie's surprise, Dr. Simon worked in the very hospital where her daughter Katarina was fighting to survive.

Desperate to help her daughter, Melanie went to see Dr. Simon, an affable man with a dark head of hair and a ready smile. He explained that in contrast to conventional wound treatment, honey bandages create a moist, clean environment. Dry scabs don't form, turning normally agonizing dressing changes into a painless routine. The honey promptly clears infection, eliminating even antibiotic-resistant bacteria. Once eliminated, the wound can progress through the normal stages of healing. Additionally, honey stimulates the secretion of cytokines,[2] which in turn stimulate the growth of new tissue at the wound edge and promote blood vessel formation to feed the growing tissue.[3]

Eager to try the new remedy, Melanie transferred Katarina into Dr. Simon's care. After swabbing Katarina's wound with Ringer solution, a sodium chloride sterile preparation, the staff applied a thin layer of medical grade honey. The wound care nurses applied fresh bandages and honey on a regular basis. The large stagnant, pus-filled wound that covered Katarina's back from a few inches below her neck to just above her anus first cleared, turning a healthy shade of red, then shrank and disappeared. Three weeks after initiating the honey treatments, Katarina's wound healed completely and required no further surgical intervention. Melanie could finally carry her daughter home.

Many of us took our good health for granted as children, stealing outside to play, run, skip, jump rope and play catch whenever the weather permitted. But for most of Dr. Simon's young patients, good health is an aspiration, the destination after a long, arduous journey through a labyrinth of hospitals, operations and bouts of chemotherapy. Traditional chemotherapy and radiation attack quickly replicating cells, suppressing the immune system and the production of new skin cells.

A suppressed immune system leaves the body open to attack; natural defenses are weakened and the body mends itself poorly. Small needle punctures, scrapes and operation scars that would normally heal quickly in a healthy child can morph into chronic, stagnant wounds. Chronic wounds invite infections. Until the sores heal, Dr. Simon must discontinue treatment. Interrupting cancer therapy gives tumors a chance to regain lost ground, a situation best avoided.

Several years ago Patrick, a twelve-year-old child, was admitted to Dr. Simon's ward at the Children's Hospital Medical Centre at the University of Bonn, Germany.[4] Prior to arriving at the clinic, doctors at another hospital partially removed an abdominal tumor, leaving an open drainage site on his stomach. Under Dr. Simon's care the wound was treated with the antibiotic Octenidin for 12 days. No improvement occurred, so Dr. Simon tested the wound and discovered a methicillin-resistant *Staphylococcus aureus* infection.

The common bacteria *Staphylococcus aureus*, known as staph, unfortunately adapts to our antibiotic use rapidly. In 1947, four short years after the first antibiotic penicillin was produced *en masse*, staph developed resistance. Doctors detected methicillin-resistant *S. aureus* (MRSA) in 1961; methicillin being the most commonly used antibiotic at the time. Our most potent antibiotic Vancomycin—reserved as the doomsday antibiotic for all resistant microorganisms—failed against staph in 2004. Swabs from three patients in an American hospital tested positive for Vancomycin resistant *S. aureus* (VRSA).

"In the United States, approximately 60 percent of staphylococcal infections in the intensive care unit are now caused by MRSA, and percentages continue to rise."[5] MRSA has spread across the globe, leaving behind a trail of destruction. In the United Kingdom, doctors battle a 70 percent MRSA wound infection rate.

In Dr. Simon's clinic, the MRSA infection rate hovers at approximately one percent. No one wanted that number to rise. It is easy to spread disease from one patient to another. It's such a common occurrence hospitals have coined a medical term to describe it: nosocomial infection, a secondary illness related to the medical intervention. To stop the resistant pathogen from spreading, Dr. Simon immediately isolated Patrick, a difficult situation for the young boy to comprehend and a managerial headache for the hospital staff.

How would they clear Patrick's infection? One of the wards intuitive wound care nurses, Ms. Blaser, had heard of the successful application of medical grade honey on resistant bacteria. She suggested the clinic try it on Patrick's infected wound.

Although Patrick was scheduled to receive multi-pronged chemotherapy, treatment could not commence until the infection cleared. Dr. Simon gave the go-ahead and after only two days of application, medical grade honey cleared the wound of MRSA. With his wound finally on the mend, Patrick started his cancer treatment on time. Since successfully treating Patrick's wound, Dr. Simon has continued to use medical grade honey in his ward with astonishing success.

---

**Nosocomial Infection:**

Hospitals have become breeding grounds for disease. Secondary illnesses acquired in a hospital and not already incubating at the time of admission to the hospital are called nosocomial infections. Estimates suggest one in ten patients in the United States picks up a nosocomial infection during a hospital stay.

Infections can also be picked up during routine outpatient medical care. To distinguish these infections the term 'health care associated infection" has been introduced.

---

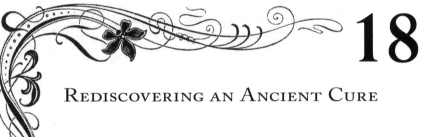

# 18

## Rediscovering an Ancient Cure

*The fruit of bees is desired by all,*
*and is equally sweet to kings and beggars*
*and it is not only pleasing but profitable and healthful;*
*it sweetens their mouths, cures their wounds,*
*and conveys remedies to inward ulcers.*

- St. Ambrose, c. 338-397

𝒲ith the skyrocketing occurrence of antibiotic resistant wound infections in hospitals, doctors grapple for solutions to pesky superbugs and rediscover the ancient use of honey. In the United Kingdom, 70 percent of staph infections in hospitals are resistant to methicillin, the most commonly used antibiotic. MRSA infections complicate and delay wound healing. Patients in UK hospitals may request wound treatment with medical honey and the National Health Service covers the cost of the prescription.[1]

Until the early 1940s, doctors frequently applied honey to wounds. When supplies ran low in China during World War II, doctors applied a mixture of honey and lard to heal ulcers, burns and small wounds.[2] The Russians used copious amounts to treat the battle wounded during World War I.[3] Surgeons cured infectious wounds with honey during the Boer War. The Greeks, Romans, Egyptians and numerous other early cultures spoke favorably of honey for wound healing. The advent of penicillin ushered in the age of antibiotics and swept honey from clinical wound care.

---

### Benefits of Honey in Wound Healing

Provides protective barrier

Prevents spreading of infection

Anti-inflammatory

Reduces swelling

Renders wound sterile

Eliminates superbugs

Diminishes pain

Rapidly eliminates wound odor

Cleans and debrides wounds

Eliminates painful surgical debridement

Promotes granulation

Stimulates new tissue growth

Improves circulation in wound bed

Moist, antibacterial wound healing environment

No pain during dressing changes

Minimizes the need for skin grafts

Helps chronic wounds pass to the next stage of healing

More rapid healing

Reduces cost and duration of medical care

Prevents scarring

Works when other traditional treatments have failed

No adverse effects

Easy to apply

Ideal dressing in remote areas, where access to medical care may be limited

Based on information provided in Molan 1999 & Lusby, Coombes et al. 2002

---

## Ancient Solution to a Modern Problem

In recent years, antibiotic resistance has forced scientists to examine alternatives to conventional wound care. "The emergence of microbial strains with multiple patterns of antimicrobial resistance has reduced the efficacy of conventional therapies and forced the re-evaluation of traditional remedies in the search for appropriate antimicrobial agents."[4]

Honey with its long record of successful application, deserves closer inspection, especially since it has proven effective against 18 strains of MRSA, seven strains of vancomycin-sensitive enterococci (VSE) and 20 strains of vancomycin-resistant enterococci (VRE) isolated from wounds or hospital environments.[5] But to understand how honey aids the healing process, we must first comprehend what happens when we sustain a wound:

"All wounds are unique, varying in size, shape, position and cause, but all wounds involve the death of epithelial cells, loss of blood, tissue damage, and the disruption of physical barriers that normally prevent infection."[6] When we puncture our skin—the largest human organ—blood pours forth, skin cells die, and our body unleashes a flood of defensive troops.

To heal, wounds must pass through three stages. The first stage involves inflammation, which permits the body to call in the repair forces. Swelling and inflammation permit greater movement of fluid and cells to the injured site. The blood clots to prevent further loss. All this rousing of the repair troops comes at a price: greater sensitivity to pain.

Usually inflammation subsides in three days, when the wound passes on to the second stage of epithelialization, the formation of new skin. Skin cells migrate across the wound bed, locking arms to form new tissue. The wound size decreases, until enough skin cells have interwoven to close the open wound. During the final maturation stage, the skin thickens to its normal strength and diminishes scar tissue.

Wounds fail to heal when they remain in the painful inflammation stage. Numerous factors contribute to a wound's inability to make the leap from inflammation to the second stage: age, diet, diabetes, immunosuppression, radiotherapy and smoking.

When injuries destroy our largest defense system—our protective skin, which makes up about 16 percent of our total body weight—the biggest foe in the battle to heal are armies of microorganisms. The most infamous bad boys of the microbial world that invade and colonize wounds are *Staphylococcus aureus*, *Pseudomonas aeruginosa*, and *Escherichia coli*.

Bacteria, which produce protein-digesting enzymes, can be very destructive to tissues. The enzymes annihilate growth factors that normally stimulate the regeneration of damaged tissue during healing.[7] Some bacteria also emit toxins that directly kill tissues.[8] Microbes have a large appetite for oxygen, stealing it away from cells that require oxygen to generate skin.[9]

Honey quickly inhibits these rabble rousers, clearing infections by eliminating the colonizing bacteria in three to 10 days.[10] New research demonstrates honey interferes with the MRSA's ability to divide and reproduce, halting the cell cycle.[11]

## Honey Stops Inflammation

Many of us have reached for a spoonful of honey to soothe a sore throat, but we probably didn't realize that its anti-inflammatory properties help a wound pass from the first to the second stage of healing. Chronic wounds that refuse to heal remain stuck in the painful inflammatory stage, unable to progress into the subsequent healing phase.

During inflammation the body sends a whole host of cells to the affected area, blood vessels dilate and surrounding areas swell. The mounting pressure restricts blood flow, "starving the tissues of oxygen and nutrients that are vital for the cells to fight infection and multiply to repair the damage"[12]. By reducing inflammation, honey improves microcirculation and increases the flow of oxygen rich blood needed for tissue repair and regeneration.

## Antioxidants And Free Radicals

Prolonged inflammation triggers the production of reactive oxygen species, known as free radicals, those unstable and dangerous molecules linked to cancer and a host of other degenerative diseases. In a wound, free radicals are bad news; they raze the essential components of functioning cells, attacking proteins, lipids and genetic material. Persistent free radical production erodes surrounding body tissues and over stimulates the production of scar tissue. This can result in "proud flesh"; an ugly mound of new tissue that sticks out from the skin surface.

Rich in antioxidants, honey scavenges for free radicals,[15] eliminating the unruly radicals before they cause trouble. By minimizing free radicals, honey suppresses painful inflammation.  Biopsies show that honey treatments reduce the number of inflammatory cells.[13,14] Flavonoids and other components of honey inhibit the creation of new free radicals in the first place.[16]

## Natural Debridement

When applied to a wound, honey soothes the swelling and reduces pain,[17] permitting the wound to pass from the inflammatory stage to regenerating new skin tissue. In this second stage, honey stimulates

---

### Microorganisms Against Which Honey Is Effective

*Methicillin-resistant Staphylococcus aureus*

*Staphylococcus aureus* (various isolates)

*Vancomycin-resistant enterococci*

*Vancomycin-sensitive enterococci* (various isolates)

*Pseudomonas aeruginosa*

*Beta-hemolytic streptococci* (various isolates)

*Alcaligenes faecalis*

*Citrobacter freundii*

*Escherichia coli*

*Enterobacter aerogenes*

*Klebsiella pneumoniae*

*Mycobacterium phlei*

*Salmonella california*

*Salmonella enteritidis*

*Salmonella typhimurium*

*Serratia marcescens*

*Shigella sonnei*

*Staphylococcus epidermidis*

*Staphylococcus capitis*

*Staphylococcus haemolyticus*

*Staphylococcus simulans*

*Staphylococcus warneri*

Information from Pieper, B. (2002). "Commentary–"Honey: a potent agent for wound healing?"." Journal of Wound, Ostomy and Continence Nursing 29: 273-274.

---

debridement, the removal of dead, damaged or infected tissue from the wound, visible as yellow, tan or black tissue. Instead of requiring painful surgical or mechanical removal, the honey dressing pulls moisture from the wound bed. This allows the tissue to release enzymes that digest and break-down dead cells; doctors call this autolytic debridement. Because the honey's osmotic action washes the wound bed from beneath, the mass of dead cells lifts off when dressings are changed.[18,19]

## TISSUE REGENERATION

Honey supports the formation of new blood vessels, and promotes wound granulation and epithelialization, the process where cells crawl across the wound bed, interlocking and weaving new skin. The army of cells regenerating new skin need energy to accomplish their work; honey provides them with the desired nutrients to proliferate. Honey wound dressings supply glucose; an energy source for the hardworking macrophages, the most important mediators of wound healing. By generating growth factors and other bioactive substances, macrophages conduct the complex process of wound healing and tissue regeneration.[20]

The amino acids in honey—proline, hydroxyproline and glycine—stimulate collagen formation and may speed the healing process.[21] Collagen provides our skin with greater elasticity[22] and strength, which is why cosmetic surgery frequently involves collagen treatments.

Evidence demonstrates honey supports our general immune system in the fight against infection. Honey inspires white blood cells to release messengers that activate our immune system response.[23] In addition to galvanizing our immune system response, lab tests confirm honey stimulates B and T cell production and activates neutrophils. All three are white blood cells responsible for identifying and killing invading bacteria and viruses.[24]

## MALODOR AND DEODORIZATION

Unfortunately many deep wounds emit foul smells, an embarrassing and depressing situation for the patient. Even before honey eliminates a wound infection, it stops the noxious odors. Bacteria munching on the amino acids from decomposed proteins in wounds produce offensive rotten egg like odors from ammonia, amines and sulfur compounds.[25] As soon as bacteria detect their preferred food glucose, which exists abundantly in honey, they quit feeding on amino acids and switch to the sugar. Since the bacteria can digest glucose without producing foul smelling waste products, the odor disappears from the wound.[26] Antibacterial honey also eliminates the odoriferous anaerobic bacteria such as *Bacteroides*, *Peptostreptococcus*, and *Prevotella* species.[27] Patients prefer honey bandages to conventional treatments because the stench of wounds from the latter curtail interactions with visitors and family and seriously impacts their quality of life.[28,29, 30]

## MOIST HEALING ENVIRONMENT

For many years doctors have known moist environments help wounds heal faster. When a scab forms, the new tissue is forced to develop underneath, leaving a pitted mar. Doctors traditionally avoid moist dressings,

---

**Wound Types that
Respond to Honey Dressings**

Abscesses

Animal wound bite

Atopic dermatitis

Burns and scalds

Herpetic lesions (lesions from Herpes)

Hidradenitis suppurativa (Acne inverse)

Infected skin-graft donor sites

Infected trauma wounds

Laceration to leg

Leg and foot ulcers

Malignant ulcers

Meningococcal septicemia skin lesions

Necrotizing fasciitis (Fournier's gangrene)

Pilonidal sinuses

Pressure ulcers

Rheumatoid ulcer

Skin grafts

Surgical wounds/infection

Traumatic wound

Tropical ulcers (Naga sores)

Based on information in Pieper 2009

---

as they offer bacteria opportunities to take up residence. Honey provides the perfect solution, a moist, yet antibacterial environment. Dry scabs don't form and the new skin remains intact during each dressing change. Traditional dressing changes often rip off the newly formed skin or dried scab, making regular dressing chances a painful and traumatic ordeal.

## REDISCOVERING THE BENEFITS OF HONEY

The beauty of honey is that in addition to stimulating wound healing, it causes no harmful or detrimental side effects. Even diabetic patients have successfully used honey dressings without raising their blood sugar levels. Occasionally patients will feel a stinging sensation, most likely caused by the acids in honey, but this is usually fleeting. It does persist in a handful of patients, yet stops immediately upon removal of the dressing. Applying a honey gel—honey mixed with wax and oil—eliminated the stinging sensation in some patients.[31]

Antibiotic drugs, in contrast, kill off good and bad bacteria. Upsetting the body's natural balance of beneficial bacteria, antibiotics can bring on diarrhea. Yeast infections can develop in the mouth, gastrointestinal tract and vagina. Antibiotics have also been linked to blood disorders, kidney stones, abnormal blood clotting, extreme sensitivity to the sun, and deafness. Occasionally antibiotics elicit allergic reactions such as a swollen face and tongue, rash, or difficulty breathing. Fatal anaphylactic reactions have also been reported.[32]

## 10 TIPS FOR HONEY APPLICATIONS[33]

- The amount of honey needed depends on the amount of fluid exuding from the wound. Wound discharge dilutes the honey. If the wound produces no exudates, the dressing should be changed twice every week. Heavily exuding wounds should be changed on a daily basis.

- Apply the honey to an absorbent dressing and then place on the wound. When you apply honey directly to the wound, it tends to run off before the dressing is applied to hold it in place.

- Honey readily soaks into absorbent bandages. By gently warming the closed honey container in a warm water bath to body temperature, or by diluting 20 parts honey to one part water, the honey will soak in more readily.

- Honey can be filled directly into cavity wounds and then covered with an adhesive film dressing, unless the wound produces large amounts of exudates.

- For moderate to heavily exuding wounds, apply a secondary bandage to contain seepage of diluted honey from the primary dressing. Polyurethane film or other types of water tight dressings are best. A secondary absorbent type dressing would draw the honey away from the wound surface and so should be avoided.

- A low-adherent dressing helps prevent the honey dressing sticking to the wound in cases where this is a problem. This dressing is placed between the wound and the honey dressing, but must be porous to allow the antibacterial components of the honey to diffuse freely into the wound bed.

- Alginate dressings impregnated with honey are a good alternative to cotton/cellulose dressings, as the alginate converts into a honey-containing soft gel.

- Fill any depressions or cavities in the wound bed with honey and then cover with a honey-impregnated dressing. This ensures the antibacterial components of the honey diffuse into the wound tissues.

- Honey can safely be inserted into any cavities or sinuses. Honey is water-soluble and easily rinsed out. Any residues are biodegradable.

- Honey dressings need to extend beyond the inflamed area surrounding a wound, since infection may lie in the tissues beyond the wound margins.

# *Interlude*

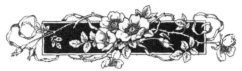

## *The Bishop and the Bees*

Saint Ambrose, the patron saint of bees, beekeepers, and candle makers, became bishop of Milan in the 4th century. Legend holds that while an infant in his cradle, a swarm of bees settled on his face, sweetening his lips with a drop of honey. An artist depicted this scene vividly on the back of the high altar of his church in Milan. People interpreted the bees kissing his infant lips with honey as a prophecy, foretelling his future as a great orator who won people over with a honeyed tongue. A similar myth accompanies the childhood of Plato:

> *when Plato was a babe the bees on Hymettus filled his mouth with honey.*[1]

As an orator, Ambrose maintained an affinity to bees, proclaiming:

> *The fruit of bees is desired by all, and is equally sweet to kings and beggars and it is not only pleasing but profitable and healthful; it sweetens their mouths, cures their wounds, and conveys remedies to inward ulcers.*[2]

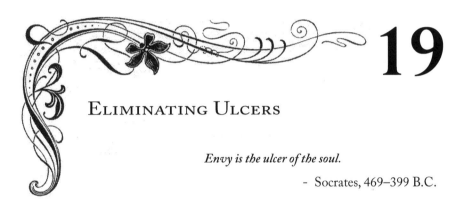

# 19

## Eliminating Ulcers

*Envy is the ulcer of the soul.*

\- Socrates, 469–399 B.C.

$\mathcal{M}$ax, a 79-year-old diabetic, developed two chronic ulcers—one on the toes and one on the heal—that refused to heal.[1] Dr. Jennifer Eddy, an associate professor of Family Medicine at the University of Wisconsin Madison, School of Medicine and Public Health and a family practitioner at Health's Family Medicine Clinic in Eau Claire, Wisconsin helped care for Max. She debrided Max's wound twice a week, removing dead tissue from the wound. With the necrotic tissue eliminated, the remaining healthy tissue would normally start to heal.

But three different strains of bacteria infected Max's ulcers: MRSA, vancomycin-resistant *Enterococcus*, and *Pseudomonas*. Max received a stringent course of antibiotics along with a diabetic shoe, which removed pressure from his foot. Despite 14 months of traditional care for chronic diabetic ulcers, his wounds refused to heal. They steadily deteriorated and he was sent to the hospital five times. He underwent four surgeries and lost two toes to gangrene as his foot turned black from lack of circulation.

Two separate surgical teams informed Max he required surgical amputation below the knee. Based on the previous complications Max suffered, the doctors offered a grim diagnosis: if he refused the amputation, he would die. Max had already been hospitalized for acute renal failure, which means his kidneys ceased functioning properly, a negative reaction to the constant flood of antibiotics.[2]

Max point blankly refused. He would rather die than have his leg removed. After speaking with the ethics committee at the hospital, the staff agreed Max had a right to choose his own treatment and he was discharged home. Max is one of 30 million patients who suffer from diabetic ulcers that are costly and difficult to treat. All together his conventional medical care cost $390,000 but failed to result in any improvement. At home and awaiting death, Max lost a third toe.

## SAVING LIVES

A family practitioner in Wisconsin, Dr. Eddy felt frustrated by Max's medical care.[3] While at the University of Massachusetts Medical School she had been a student in Dr. Guido Majno's class, who spent over 10 years writing *The Healing Hand: Man and the Wound in the Ancient World*. She distinctly recalled how her professor insisted honey was the most effective ancient remedy for wounds. In his book, Majno describes the benefits of honey:

> *The swnw* (physician) *happened to choose an ingredient that was practically harmless to the tissues, aseptic, antiseptic, and an antibiotic. I should say the ingredient: nothing else, in ancient Egypt, could have begun to match these properties of honey.*[4]

Dr. Eddy read up on healing with honey and then approached the infectious disease coordinator at the hospital where she practiced. Since Max had refused amputation and nothing else was working, the hospital granted permission to try honey.

"I wasn't very optimistic to begin with," Dr. Eddy said during an interview, "which is why I didn't photograph his foot ulcers right away. Within two to three weeks his ulcers had improved so much, I started taking pictures to document his recovery. Then the nurses applying the honey said it was non-standard care and so they couldn't continue implementing it."

By the time the nurses refused to continue, the evidence of healing spoke for itself. Max's wife offered to apply the honey dressings herself. She purchased ordinary honey from the supermarket. Every day she poured a thick coating of honey onto 4" x 4" gauze pads, which she then placed on her husband's ulcers. The honey proved so effective, Max's orally administered antibiotics and saline dressings were discontinued.

Granulation tissue, the dark pink bumpy new skin that marks the first signs of healing, appeared two weeks after starting the honey dressings. Three months passed and the ulcer on the heel reduced in size to a small dimple. By six months it healed completely. The ulcer on the front of his foot where Max lost three toes to gangrene took twelve months to heal completely.

Two years have since passed and the ulcers on Max's foot didn't reappear. He can now move on his own with the assistance of a walker and enjoys a tremendous increase in his quality of life. According to his original prognosis he should be dead, but he's walking thanks to Dr. Eddy's intervention with honey.

Dr. Eddy rightly feels proud of her work. For her, the most important factor is a good patient outcome. Currently she is recruiting diabetic foot ulcer patients in Wisconsin for a controlled double-blind study comparing off the shelf supermarket honey with a placebo that looks and smells like honey.

Worldwide 200 million people suffer from diabetes. In the United States 18.8 million have been diagnosed with diabetes.[5] Much more alarmingly, over seven million Americans have diabetes but don't know it because they have never been tested. At some point in their life, 15-25 percent of all diabetics develop an ulcer, so the U.S. must grapple with up to 6.3 million ulcers.

The costs for treating diabetic ulcers are high. Max's care alone cost $390,000. It's not hard to see how the United States spent $10.9 billion on diabetic ulcer care in 2001. Medical care costs continue to rise as does the number of people with diabetes. Honey bandages of diabetic ulcers could help us reign in some of those escalating costs.

According to an article published in the *New York Times*, diabetes is a silent epidemic.

*"How bad is the diabetes epidemic?" asked Frank Vinicor,*
*associate director for public health practice at the Centers for Disease*

*Control. "There are several ways of telling. One might be how many different occurrences in a 24-hour period of time, between when you wake up in the morning and when you go to sleep. So, 4,100 people diagnosed with diabetes, 230 amputations in people with diabetes, 120 people who enter end-stage kidney disease programs and 55 people who go blind.*

*"That's going to happen every day, on the weekends and on the Fourth of July," he said. "That's diabetes."*[6]

In 2000-2001 diabetics underwent 82,000 amputations of lower limbs.[7] Diabetes claims more limbs than any other ailment; 60 percent of all non-traumatic amputations in the U.S. are performed on diabetics. Diabetics typically first lose a toe, then another, until eventually the whole foot must come off. The lack of circulation causes the wound to stagnate and gangrene sets in. To save the patient's life, doctors amputate the leg. The loss of a limb severely reduces both the individual's and family's quality of life. Restricted in movement, the amputee can do less and requires more help from family members or caregivers. Good health care and a multidisciplinary team of experts significantly reduce the chances of losing a limb.

"I'm a primary care provider in the real world," Dr. Eddy said. "Many diabetics have limited access to wound care specialists. Simple honey on gauze *can* have a significant impact."

Compared to typical diabetic prescriptions, supermarket honey is a cheap alternative. "There are strong economic disincentives for researching honey," Dr. Eddy explained. "One of my patients used to be on Regranex˚." Dr. Eddy quickly pointed out she wasn't knocking Regranex, an immune system booster that contains a platelet derived growth factor. Growth factors signal the body has sustained an injury and the repair troops should come in to fix it. The growth factor is supposed to throw the body from a chronic wound back into the first stages of an acute wound and so stimulate the healing process. "The Regranex˚ treatment costs my patient $1,000 per month. Companies selling that won't want to hear 43¢ of honey and gauze is just as effective."

When Dr. Eddy first tried to publish her case study results, she was very optimistic that the research journals would be interested in her findings. After all Max's medical care had cost $390,000 and failed to work. A few hundred dollars worth of honey and gauze had healed the ulcers completely, saving Max from an amputation. An accomplished writer, Dr.

Eddy submitted her paper to highly respected journals such as the *Lancet* and the *Journal of the American Medical Association* (JAMA). One of the reviewers for JAMA turned down the paper, because he didn't see the significance of the cost of prior treatment.

"I've become much more cynical about the medical profession since then," Dr. Eddy said. But she's not letting naysayers stop her important work. She feels she's ethically required to inform patients of the possibility of honey when confronted with chronic wounds. Always wanting the best for her patients, she carefully explains her previous experiences and lets them decide if it's appropriate on their own.

---

**The UK National Health Service Bulletin
lists the following benefits of honey dressings:[8]**

Potent antibacterial agent

Effective against a range of multi-resistant organisms

Promotes environment that promotes autolytic debridement

Bacteria prefer sugar to protein, so metabolic product is lactic acid, as opposed to more malodorous compounds

Stimulates granulation tissue

Anti-inflammatory activity

Effectiveness noticeable when conventional antimicrobials (antibiotics/antiseptics) have failed

No adherence to wound bed

---

## A Second Chance: Venous Leg Ulcers

Honey works well with diabetic ulcers, as exemplified by Dr. Eddy's treatment of Max. The two most common types of leg ulcers are venous and arterial ulcers. As the names suggest, arterial ulcers occur from blocked arteries, while venous ulcers involve blocked veins. Arteries carry oxygenated blood from our heart to our extremities, while veins carry the oxygen-deprived blood back to the heart.

Because the arteries handle blood being pumped from the heart under high pressure, they are thick and elastic. Veins, in contrast, have a thin, elastic muscle layer with valves that stop the deoxygenated blood from flowing backward.

When an individual suffers from inadequate circulation of blood, arterial ulcers develop. These wounds usually occur on the lower third of the leg, especially in-between toes, on the shin or outside ankle, or over pressure points. The wounds are typically circular and deep with smooth edges, like an abscess. No swelling accompanies these painful ulcers. Due to lack of circulation, the skin feels cool to the touch.

Venous ulcers form when high pressure in the veins causes them to compress or collapse. The one-way valves in veins ensure that the blood flows from superficial veins—a fine network of veins located between the skin and muscle—to the deep veins located between muscles. The flexing of our calf muscles as we walk provides the power to drive the blood back up the leg. The one-way valves prevent backflow, so when the muscle relaxes, the now empty vein can refill again with blood from the superficial veins.

When pressure builds up, these valves can malfunction, allowing blood to flow in the wrong direction from the deep veins back out to the superficial ones. This backflow causes congestion and the failure of more valves. Blood escapes and leaks through the vessel walls into surrounding tissues. Clots form to stop the blood flow and tissues die off. Typically irregular in shape and shallow, venous ulcers look very different from arterial ulcers. The most common symptom is swelling, accompanied by dry, flaky skin with blotchy discoloration or eczema.

About two percent of all adults suffer from venous leg ulcers, which are slow to heal. Doctors prescribe compression therapy, tight four-layer bandages that constrict swelling and backflow of blood, to alleviate venous ulcers.

Sadly intervention only works in 32-50 percent of all venous ulcers. Those that do heal, typically half reoccur within three months.[9] It's not uncommon for patients to experience two to ten episodes of ulceration or for ulcers to last more than 18 months.[10]

Chronic wounds often support four or more pathogens. Such infections delay healing, accentuate wound size and can lead to life-threatening illness. Worst-case scenarios include amputation and even death.

The first step in healing chronic ulcers is wound debridement, the removal of necrotic tissue and slough, the yellowish mass of dead cells. Dr. Georgina Gethin and Dr. Seamus Cowman from the Royal College of Surgeons in Ireland study the effects of honey on wound debridement in venous leg ulcers.

Their initial interest was piqued by the fantastic response of chronic ulcers under their care to honey dressings. In 2005 they published a report about eight patients whose wounds had not shown any signs of improvement to at least four weeks of traditional wound care.[11]

Vincent, an 82-year-old man, had suffered from a venous ulcer for the last 18 months.[12] His wound, a 3.75 $cm^2$ opening, languished and refused to heal. Non-responding wounds often leave patients disinterested in their health outcome. Nothing seems to help, so they feel frustrated and powerless.

Vincent's wound responded immediately to the honey dressings, shrinking by 25 percent in the first week. "Unlike many modern wound dressings, honey acts intimately with the wound environment and has the ability to connect directly with all surfaces not just the more superior wound surfaces," the doctors noted in their report.[13]

When Vincent saw his wound respond to the honey treatment, his doctors noted increased self-interest and compliance with his wound care. During the four weeks of honey treatment, Vincent's wound was dressed once or twice weekly with five grams (approximately 1 teaspoon) of manuka honey on non-adherent gauze. Honey works when other conventional treatments have failed. Although Vincent's wound had not improved during 18 months of conventional treatment, four weeks of honey dressings shrank his wound by 86 percent. By the end of the four week trial, all that remained was a tiny 0.50 $cm^2$ opening.

The honey dressings worked well for all patients, whose average wound size decreased by almost 55 percent. Malodor vanished from all wounds; a welcome relief to patients and family members.

Two patients that suffered from insufficient circulation reported a stinging sensation in response to the honey treatments. Their wounds improved minimally, perhaps suggesting that honey may be less effective in arterial ulcers that suffer from lack of blood flow.

## HONEY VS. HYDROGEL IN VENOUS LEG ULCERS

Intrigued by their initial findings Drs. Gethin and Cowman launched a large, randomized control study comparing manuka honey dressings to standard hydrogel therapy in more than a hundred patients.[14] Ten different sites, including hospitals and ulcer clinics, recruited patients with sloughy, venous leg ulcers from 2003 until 2006. For an individual to be included in the study the ulcer had to be less than 100 cm² and at least half of it had to be covered with slough at time of enrollment.

To control for potential bias, patients were blindly assigned to receive either five grams of manuka honey or three grams of hydrogel per 20 cm² bandage (the difference in volume between treatments made up for the disparity in viscosity). In addition to the honey or hydrogel treatment, patients continued normal compression therapy, typically a four-layer bandage.

The dressings were refreshed on a weekly basis for four weeks. Prior to each dressing change, wound care specialists cleaned the tissue with warm tap water. Wounds were evaluated at four weeks and again after twelve weeks to monitor their progression. After four weeks, 80 percent of the wounds had lost more than half of the slough in response to both treatments, however new tissue growth appeared more rapidly in wounds treated with manuka honey.

More interestingly, the manuka treated wounds shrank by 34 percent compared to only 13 percent in hydrogel treated wounds. Dr. Gethin believes one reason honey treatments work so well in chronic wounds is because they lower the pH of the wound. Chronic wounds typically boast an alkaline environment, which favors the build-up of necrotic tissue. This additional slough in turn promotes a bacteria-friendly environment. The bacteria feed on the slough and release ammonia waste products, which further deteriorate the wound. The scarred tissue and poor vasculature of chronic and recurrent wounds like venous ulcers hinder the transport of oxygen, arresting wound recovery.

Honey dressings lower wound pH, which stimulates increased oxygen release, destruction of abnormal wound collagen and new blood vessel formation. Dr. Gethin found that a reduction in pH of 0.1 units correlated with an 8.1 percent reduction in wound size.[15] Compared to hydrogel therapy, manuka dressings increased the rates of healing, cleared necrotic tissue more effectively and resulted in lower wound infection rates of venous leg ulcers. Having stood up to the rigor of a randomized trial, manuka wound dressings have demonstrated their effectiveness in modern wound management.

Another larger randomized clinical trial compared Apinate dressings, a manuka honey impregnated dressing, to standard care to see if honey exerted an additional benefit to venous ulcer healing beyond compression therapy alone.[16] The 368 patients recruited between May 2004 and September 2005, were followed for 12 weeks. At that time 55.6 percent of the ulcers receiving the honey bandages healed completely compared to 49.7 percent of the ulcers treated with standard care. The wounds shrank 74.1 percent with honey versus 65.5 percent with conventional therapy. Only 37 patients receiving honey dressings developed wound infections compared to 49 from conventional treatment. When all costs were considered, the honey dressings proved more cost-effective. While the authors concluded that honey did not exert a statistically significant benefit over compression therapy, those treated with honey did have higher healing rates, less infections and were less costly to treat.

## MEDIHONEY AND VENOUS LEG ULCERS

Registered nurse Cheryl Dunford, a faculty member in House Sciences at Southampton University in the United Kingdom, also looked at how venous leg ulcers responded to honey dressings.[17] The wounds of 40 participants had all failed to respond to 12 weeks of conventional compression therapy at the time of enrollment in her study, which recruited patients from November 2001 until August 2002. Their treatment regime was not changed except for the addition of approximately 20g of Medihoney—an active medical honey blend—to a 10 x 10 cm sterile bandage.

Unfortunately 13 patients dropped out of the study due to increased pain, impaired health or wound deterioration, although the deterioration was not caused by the honey. While pain levels increased in some patients, none of the patients who dropped out reported any pain during dressing changes with honey.

Pain dominates the lives of many with leg ulcers and patients frequently have other health issues. Many individuals who live with venous leg ulcers find conventional treatments agonizing and so don't comply with wound care instructions. When an ulcer patient was questioned about her non-compliance for a survey on living with venous leg ulcers, she responded: "I just kept telling the nurse it was too painful …but she insisted it was the right treatment … After she left I took it all off."[18] Interestingly, the Medihoney bandages reduced the level of pain felt by half of the patients.

For those who still work, the difficulty of managing their wounds can be overwhelming. One individual recounted his troubles hiding his embarrassing wound exudates at work:

> *"Used to try all sorts but in the end wore wellington* (rain) *boots at work … anything to hide the leakage."[19]*

Malodor seriously impacts the lives of those living with chronic wounds. "I've known many patients, who stopped socializing, became very embarrassed, stopped going out," Cheryl Dunford explained.[20]

In a study on how ulcers impact people's daily lives, one individual offered this insight about how her wound odor changed her life:

> The odor has been unbearable ... I used to go to church, but the person next to me could smell my leg ... so I don't go now.[21]

"It has a very demoralizing effect on patients," Cheryl Dunford explained. "Yet it's an area where nurses are reluctant to question patients ... Patients are often embarrassed to discuss this." One of the major benefits of the honey dressings is the rapid decrease in wound malodor. In Dunford's venous leg trial, the patients attributed the substantial drop off in wound odor to the new honey dressings.

The patients who remained in the study for the 12 week duration all experienced reduced wound size and swelling. Seven individuals watched with joy as their ulcers healed completely.

Vivian, an eighty-five-year-old lady, had struggled with her right leg for 20 months.[22] Numerous small ulcers dotted her shin. Fit and otherwise healthy, she attended a local leg ulcer clinic every week, where nurses changed the dressing beneath her compression bandage.

Small, inflexible, white calcium deposits formed in her leg, whose irregular shape could be traced on her skin. They sat firmly entrenched in the wound bed of her ulcers, hampering recovery. The calcium deposits kept the tissue inflamed, so the ulcers never shrank in size despite regular care.

Once every three months Vivian travelled to a vascular clinic, where the staff surgically removed each individual calcium deposit - a painful and anxiety ridden procedure that caused her ulcers to bleed. But Vivian knew it needed to be done, otherwise the individual deposits would fuse into larger pieces.

Registered nurse Cheryl Dunford met Vivian while recruiting patients for her venous leg ulcer clinical trial.[23] The petite woman agreed to try the manuka honey impregnated dressings. During the very first dressing change, the staff noted that pieces of calcium clung to the honey bandage. With each passing week, the honey dressings pulled out additional deposits, naturally debriding the wound without painful surgical intervention. Vivian naturally loved the honey dressings, as she no longer needed to attend the agonizing sessions at the vascular clinic every three months.

Poor health conditions dictate that some individuals will contend with life-long leg ulcerations, regardless of treatment. Honey dressings can improve a person's quality of life by reducing pain and eliminating odor, even if complete healing lies beyond their reach.

## Pressure Ulcers And Retirement Homes

As we age, we become more prone to injuring ourselves. The years roll by; our skin dries out, loses its elasticity and the nourishing blood supply diminishes. This leaves elderly individuals prone to injury. Once wounded, the healing process creeps forward slowly. Tears in the skin and areas under pressure require constant vigilance or else they deteriorate quickly.

In nursing homes, the staff is often overworked. Daily dressing changes are costly and problematic, especially when patients resist care. According to registered nurse Elizabeth van der Weyden of the Wood-field Retirement Village in New South Wales, Australia, "What is needed in many settings caring for older people is a dressing that can provide an antimicrobial base, reduce inflammation, odor, pain, reduce the frequency of dressing changes and is easy to apply and remove."[24]

She discovered the perfect solution - Apinate, an alginate dressing impregnated with medical grade honey. Alginate dressings, made from a seaweed component, interact with fluids in the wound to create a gel-like substance. Highly absorbent, these bandages generate a moist wound environment that promotes healing.

Robert spent many of his 83 years working outside. Harsh sun exposure during earlier years had deteriorated his skin, leaving it prone to wounds.[25] Mildly obese, Robert suffered from transient ischemic attacks (TIA), which resemble the symptoms of stroke but cause no brain damage. When they struck, Robert experienced sudden weakness and paralysis on the right side of his body, slurred speech and dizziness. As an aftereffect, his right ankle tended to lean toward his right side, creating a pressure area. A sore developed rapidly, escalating into an ulcer in a few days.

Traditional wound treatment for three weeks with hydrocolloid, gel-forming bandages brought no signs of healing. Frustrated at Robert's lack of progress, Elizabeth van der Weyden sought approval from his doctor and wife to apply the honey-impregnated alginate dressing. When granted, she washed his ankle to remove remnants of the old dressing, cleansed it with saline and then applied the Apinate bandage to his ankle. To absorb wound exudates, she placed a cotton pad on top of the honey dressing. Then to hold everything in place, she applied a cotton tubular bandage around his ankle.

Initially she replaced the dressing twice per week, as the wound gave off a slight odor. The wound showed signs of healing within the first week. By the thirteenth day, the wound odor disappeared. Within six weeks, the wound shrunk to half its size and new tissue growth could be seen. The ulcer healed completely in 11 weeks and Robert regained complete use of his foot.

Guido arrived at Woodfield Retirement Village after a two week hospital stay.[26] Born in Italy during the First World War, 84-year-old Guido suffered from very poor health—chronic back pain coupled with Parkinson's disease and dementia—which left him frail and virtually immobile.

Doctors had previously performed prostate surgery—known as a transurethral resection of the prostate or TURP—to relieve the painful blockage of the urinary track caused by his enlarged prostate. At his most recent hospitalization he received treatment for his recurrent urinary tract infection and lower back pain.

A painful pressure ulcer covered Guido's lower back, right above the anus. The hospital had discharged him with a large piece of hydrocolloid dressing over the wound. When the staff at Woodfield removed the dressing, they found a small festering and necrotic area surrounded by tender, inflamed skin. Guido winced when nurses touched the area.

Nurses cleaned the wound with saline and then applied SoloSite gel and a hydrocolloid dressing to encourage wound debridement as recommended by Guido's hospital discharge papers. SoloSite creates and maintains a moist wound environment, which encourages natural wound debridement. Ideally the necrotic tissue will loosen and then lift off with normal dressing changes.

However, due to the awkward location of the ulcer just above the buttocks, the hydrocolloid gel-forming dressing refused to stay in place. The staff switched to another gel product on a low-adherent absorbent pad, which they held in place with tape. Four weeks of treatment brought no improvement to Guido's wound - the hard, necrotic tissue refused to break down and the inflammation continued unabated, leaving him in agony.

Elizabeth van der Weyden decided to switch his care over to an Apinate dressing, believing the honey's tendency to reduce inflammation and stimulate self-debridement would benefit poor Guido. His wound was gently cleansed with saline and then a 5 x 3 cm Apinate bandage applied to the pressure ulcer.

His wound responded immediately to the honey dressing. The hard scab disintegrated, revealing a deep pus-filled opening extremely painful to the touch. During the second week, the wound care nurse removed the outer dressing and showered the area to cleanse it. The warm water of the shower caused the inner honey alginate dressing to lift off easily, simultaneously debriding the wound. The honey had softened the hard wound surface, allowing it to naturally lift off with the dressing change. Another week of honey dressings and Guido's necrotic tissue all but disappeared. New tissue growth surrounded the edges of the wound bed.

By the fifth week, the ulcer shrank to half its original size; healthy tissue surrounded the wound. Guido's inflammation had evaporated, making dressing changes much less painful. By the following week, the wound had split into two small dime sized areas. Two months after starting the honey alginate dressings, Guido's lower back had healed completely, leaving behind no scars.

Since Robert and Guido's excellent outcomes, the staff at Woodfield Retirement Village successfully treated numerous other chronic wounds with honey-impregnated alginate dressings. Instead of gravitating toward Apinate dressings when other treatments fail, the staff now routinely uses Apinate dressings to treat the wounds of their elderly patients.[27]

## Pressure Ulcers: Antibiotics or Honey

Two doctors in Izmir, Turkey, Dr. Ülkü Yapucu Güneş and Dr. Ismet Eşer from the Ege University School of Nursing, found the growing body of research on honey intriguing.[28] They were curious to learn whether pressure ulcers responded better to honey dressings or a topical antibiotic treatment.

Before starting their study, they were convinced the honey dressings would prove no more effective than topical applications of ethoxy-diaminoacridine and nitrofurazone, an antibiotic combination used with great success in contaminated wounds throughout Turkey. To see if they were right, they recruited 26 patients with 50 pressure ulcers on the shoulder, the sacrum (base of the spine), at the trochanters (bony area of hip where muscles attach), or the heel.

Patients were randomly assigned to the two treatment groups. Fifteen individuals with 25 pressure ulcers received daily applications of raw, unpasteurized honey that had been gamma-irradiated to remove all potential spores. Prior to application, the honey was tested to ensure it had a high level of antibacterial activity. The doctors then washed the wounds with a 0.9 percent sodium-chloride solution and applied a bandage soaked with approximately 20 ml of honey, ensuring it made full contact with the open ulcer. To stop wound leakage, a semi-permeable adhesive dressing was applied on top. Patients received daily dressing changes; each time the wound was first rinsed with sodium-chloride solution. As soon as the wounds were dry and clean the doctors decreased the frequency of dressing changes to every other day.

The 11 patients in the control group also had 25 pressure ulcers. The doctors first cleaned the ulcers with a 0.1 percent ethoxy-diaminoacridine solution, then spread the nitrofurazone cream on the wound surface. Finally they covered the ulcer with gauze soaked in the ethoxy-diaminoacridine solution. An additional semi-permeable adhesive dressing served as a secondary bandage, just as it did in the honey group. Dressings were changed daily during the five week trial.

The most rigorous clinic trials are blinded, which means the doctor doesn't know what treatment a patient receives when he evaluates the patient's progress. Although Dr. Güneş and Dr. Eşer would have preferred a blinded trial, the nature of the treatments made this impossible. Each wound would require rinsing with sodium-chloride immediately before the wound was evaluated for progress, so the assessor couldn't see traces of the treatment. But such rinsing would disturb the wound bed, removing slough and wound exudates and eliminate all possibility of an accurate assessment of wound progression.

To their surprise, Dr. Güneş and Dr. Eşer discovered that while the pressure ulcers in both groups improved, patients treated with honey dressings showed four times the rate of healing compared to the antibiotic group. Honey treated pressure ulcers contracted by 56 percent, versus a 13 percent reduction in the other patients. While no ulcers healed completely with five weeks of antibiotic dressings, 20 percent of the honey treated ulcers disappeared.

"Honey (is) an attractive treatment option for topical management of pressure ulcers," the doctors concluded.[29] Pressure ulcers and bedsores occur commonly in bedridden and elderly patients. Mounting evidence confirms the effectiveness of honey dressings to heal such stubborn wounds.

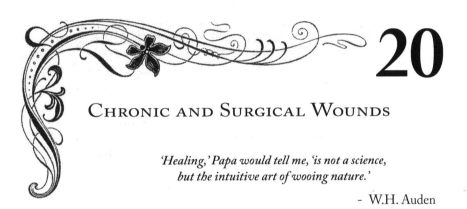

# 20

## CHRONIC AND SURGICAL WOUNDS

*'Healing,' Papa would tell me, 'is not a science,*
*but the intuitive art of wooing nature.'*

- W.H. Auden

$K$atrien, a 75-year-old woman,[1] suffered from rheumatoid arthritis and vasculitis; an inflammation of the blood vessels.[2] For over four years, the extensive, foul-smelling wounds on both her legs deteriorated despite continuous care. To counteract the inflammation of her rheumatoid arthritis, her doctors prescribed high daily doses of prednisolone. But such corticosteroid medications suppress the immune system. Without a fully functioning immune system, wounds heal poorly. Katrien's legs looked as though they had gone through a meat grinder; they rotted away as she watched on helplessly.

Frustrated by her stagnating and odoriferous wounds, a team of medical doctors in Amsterdam decided to try honey dressings on her legs. Although her wounds had not responded to four years of traditional treat-

171

ment, the foul stench disappeared almost immediately when dressed with honey. Within three weeks the wounds showed granulation with islands of new skin formation.

Chest pain and frequent shortness of breath sent 63-year-old Jacco to seek the advice of his doctor.[3] Upon closer examination, a heart specialist determined Jacco had a blocked artery leading to his heart. He needed coronary bypass surgery.

A team of specialists cut a long incision into the skin of Jacco's calf and carefully harvested a section of his great saphenous vein, the large vein running the length of his leg. Doctors prefer to use a section of this healthy vein to divert blood flow around the heart's blocked artery. The heart specialists then successfully connected the harvested vein, rerouting and restoring normal blood flow to the heart muscles.

Although the bypass surgery went smoothly, the long 17 x 2 cm gash on Jacco's calf refused to heal. The wound care nurses applied highly absorbent calcium alginate dressings on a daily basis, but the surgical incision stagnated. His doctors decided to switch him to honey dressings, which jump started the wound healing process. Six weeks of honey dressings and Jacco's leg healed completely.

Katrien and Jacco were two of the original 13 patients treated by a medical team of four doctors in the Netherlands. Burn experts or plastic and reconstructive surgeons, the four Dutch doctors implemented honey dressing when their patients' wounds failed to respond to a multitude of traditional treatments including calcium alginate dressings, silver sulfadiazine bandages, zinc oxide ointment, hydrocolloid polymer dressing, or vacuum-assisted closure. Instead of improving the wounds, these conventional remedies exacerbated the size of some.

During the initial three months, the team gained experience in using the honey dressings on complex cases. The initial 13 patients responded favorably to the honey-dressings, so the team of doctors expanded their study to include 60 patients, whose wounds had failed to heal with conventional therapy.

The 60 patients, treated between June 2000 and June 2001, fell into one of three groups: 21 with chronic wounds, 23 with complicated surgical wounds and 16 with acute traumatic wounds. All of the wounds were rinsed with a saline solution and then covered with the honey impregnated dressing on a daily basis. Treatment lasted anywhere from one to 28 weeks, depending on the nature of the wound.

All but one patient, who dropped out due to pain, completed the study. Of the 59 remaining patients, 57 attained full wound healing and the wounds of the remaining two patients did not deteriorate. The four doctors noted that the wounds responded favorably to the honey dressings, which decreased swelling and wound exudates, enhanced debridement, decreased odor and hastened the formation of new skin tissue. The Dutch experts believe honey-impregnated dressings make "a useful addition to the armamentarium for the management of chronic and acute wounds".[4] Armamentarium is the equipment, methods, and pharmaceuticals used in medicine.

When flummoxed by a wound that won't respond to any conventional treatment, doctors appear willing to try a promising, new remedy. Honey has proven so effective under these worst case scenarios that many once skeptical wound care professionals now routinely implement honey dressings for wound care.

## CHRONIC WOUNDS RESPOND TO HONEY DRESSINGS

Honey impregnated tulle dressings proved effective in managing 20 chronic wounds from July to October, 2003 in the United Kingdom that did not respond to traditional therapies. Jackie Stephen-Haynes, a lecturer and practitioner in Tissue Viability for Worcester Primary Care Trusts and University College Worcester, evaluated Activation Tulle, a honey based wound dressing available in the United Kingdom.[5]

Henrietta, an 88-year-old blind and wheelchair bound woman suffered from osteoarthritis and chronic leg ulcers that continued to deteriorate under conventional therapy.[6] Her wheelchair had been her only form of mobility for 30 years. Frustrated with the lack of progress, she didn't always comply with the doctor's recommendations to elevate her legs and continue her medications. High compression bandages and other conventional therapies she'd tried over the years proved ineffective in reducing her leg ulcerations, which continued to decline. The skin around the large ulcers swelled and became inflamed.

An MRI scan revealed Henrietta required surgery to repair artery damage in her legs. Blocked arteries stopped sufficient blood flow to her extremities. A team of doctors performed angioplasty in both her legs, successfully widening the blocked artery in her left leg. Intervention in her right leg proved less effective.

The tissues surrounding her ulcers started to breakdown and swell, in part because Henrietta didn't keep her legs elevated as instructed nor regularly take her prescribed diuretics, both of which reduce swelling.

Discouraged by wound stagnation, many individuals like Henrietta lose interest in their chronic wound care and so fail to comply with doctor recommendations.

Always hopeful, Henrietta agreed to try the new honey impregnated Activation Tulle dressings. Her legs stung as the honey made contact. The stinging sensation continued throughout the first night and Henrietta slept fitfully. But she was determined to see this through. When the dressings were changed the next day, the stinging sensation decreased significantly and disappeared half an hour later.

Henrietta watched her legs improve rapidly. She could finally see progress and now complied with the doctor's request to keep her legs elevated and take her prescribed medications. Four weeks later, the macerated skin surrounding the wound had healed completely. The leg ulcers showed signs of new tissue growth and Henrietta was well on her way to full recovery.

Angela, despite her 88 years, was sprightly and enjoyed full use of her legs.[7] One day she lost her balance and fell into an electric fire, burning her upper left arm. Doctors left the wound to dry out. A tough, thick eschar formed on the 15 x 20 cm wound.

To encourage the thick, dry necrotic mass of tissue to fall off, her wound care team applied hydrogel bandages. This type of dressing creates a moist environment, which is supposed to promote debridement of the necrotic scab. Despite the hydrogel treatment, the wound stayed dry and painful. A swab showed MRSA had colonized Angela's arm. The doctors put her on two antibiotics: amoxicillin and flucloxacillin.

Angela found the hydrogel dressings and antibiotic treatments distressing. The scab remained dry, leaving the wound tight and painful. When her burn wound showed no sign of improvement after one and a half weeks, they asked her if she wanted to try the new honey dressings. The wound care team explained the dressing should stimulate autolysis and then the scab would lift off. Angela consented and the hydrogel dressings were swapped out for the Activation Tulle.

Within one week, the honey dressings softened the hard eschar, turning it from a dark blackish brown to a golden yellow. The softer scab alleviated the tightness in the burn, bringing welcome relief from pain. By week three the wound debrided itself and after ten weeks of honey dressings, new tissue growth was visible at the burn site. Angela, pleased with the fast progress, remarked that the dressings were comfortable and convenient to wear. She never experienced any pain during dressing changes.

The two elderly women, Henrietta and Angela, were among 18 patients whose chronic wounds responded favorably to honey impregnated dressings. Two additional patients showed no improvement, but their wounds did not deteriorate further. It is remarkable that 80 percent responded well when their wounds had failed to show signs of healing using conventional wound care. All of the individuals Jackie Stephen-Haynes followed suffered from sloughy wounds that gave off offensive odors prior to the honey dressings.

From evaluation forms the patients and nurses completed, she learned that 65 percent considered the dressing easy to apply, while 30 percent found the ease of dressing changes to be on par with prior treatments. Only one patient found it more difficult, most likely because the honey dressing size was too large to easily wrap around his small wound.

Three-quarters felt the honey dressings were easily removed, while the remaining quarter responded they were average. Dressing changes of chronic wounds are notoriously difficult. Many standard dressings adhere to the wound bed, making removal traumatic and painful. Honey dressings in contact with an exudating wound are essentially in a fluid state. The dressing can thus be lifted off without sticking. Any excess honey is simply rinsed away, before a new dressing is placed on the wound.

Such positive outcomes from chronic wounds that failed to respond to conventional therapy warrant that honey dressings should be "an additional effective wound management product rather than an alternative to existing treatments".[8]

## THE HEALING TOUCH OF HONEY

A short walk from the bustling market square in the city center of Bonn, the former capital of Germany, sits a corpulent yet demure old villa with a broad steep flight of stairs. The occasional arrival of an ambulance into its long circular drive hints that this otherwise quiet corner is part of the University Clinic of Bonn.

Step inside and you are greeted by a sizeable jungle gym in bright cheery primary colors and several sturdy wooden animals on top of thick, bouncy metal springs. A young child playfully rocks back and forth on top of a horse, oblivious to the doctors in white coats whizzing past.

This is the clinic of Dr. Arne Simon, who you met in the introduction to Part III. With the help of his wound care specialist nurse Ms.

Blaser, he eliminated MRSA from Patrick's stomach wound and cleared the nasty back infection of the newborn Katarina. Since treating Patrick with Medihoney in 2002, Dr. Simon and his team continue to implement honey on chronic wounds with astounding success. In addition to Patrick, they treated six adults, who ranged from 42 to 66 years of age. All of them had chronic wounds infected with MRSA,[9] wounds sustained during surgery in all but one case.

Sebastian, a 42-year-old diabetic, had undergone coronary bypass surgery to improve blood flow to his heart.[10] After surgery he developed a nasty MRSA wound infection along two of the incisions doctors had cut into his chest. Such sternal wound infections are an uncommon but potentially life-threatening complication of cardiac surgery.

While recovering from the operation, MRSA then invaded his lungs, causing life-threatening MRSA pneumonia. To fight the resistant infection, the doctors put Sebastian on systemic antibiotics, flooding his system with vancomycin to try and halt the deadly disease.

The festering wounds on his chest were treated with povidone-iodine. The bones in his chest became infected from the bacteria, what doctors call osteomyelitis. His wounds leaked thick, yellowish pus with a pungent, foul odor.

For 360 days Sebastian battled unsuccessfully against the chest wound infections. Despite constant antibiotics, the MRSA infection continued. To alleviate the long suffering Sebastian, the doctors then switched him over to Medihoney Antibacterial Medical Honey during his outpatient care. The open cavity was filled with Medihoney and then a calcium alginate dressing placed on top to keep the honey in contact with the wound.

When doctors took their next swab from his chest a hundred days later, it was clear. The MRSA infection had been eradicated and Sebastian's wounds were finally on their way to healing. Because of all the complications and Sebastian's poor health, his surgical wound healed slowly.

Sebastian and the other six patients liked the Medihoney wound treatment. It cleansed the wound and stimulated healing, which encouraged them to cooperate in their wound care. Despite the regular use of antiseptics for wound care in all patients and systemic treatment with vancomycin antibiotics in three, the MRSA infections had stubbornly refused to clear under conventional care. One patient tried to eliminate the MRSA infection unsuccessfully for five years before switching to the honey dressings, which efficiently controlled the MRSA colonization.

While the ancient Egyptians and Greeks used honey for wound care, Medihoney is the first medically certified honey in Europe. Despite its effectiveness in wound care, Medihoney is not certified as medicine in the European Union (EU) but as a medical device, defined as "any instrument, apparatus, appliance, material or other article …to be used for … the purpose of diagnosis, prevention, monitoring, treatment or alleviation of disease."[11] This puts Medihoney on par with thermometers, bandages, silver dressings, or crutches.

Because Medihoney has received certification in the EU, it can be prescribed by a dermatologist or general physician, in which case medical insurance must cover the cost. It is also available over the counter from pharmacies and online, but without a prescription, the buyer bears the brunt of the cost.

The FDA approved Medihoney in the United States in June 2007. Derma Sciences, an American wound care company manufactures the U.S. product for the Australian based company Comvita. They rolled out Medihoney alginate wound dressings in November, 2007. Pure medical honey in a tube as used at the Bonn clinic is now also available.

When asked if he would recommend Medihoney for use in the home against scrapes, burns or cuts, Dr. Simon responded with an affirmative. Medihoney has a place in every medicine cabinet. Having learned of his successful use of Medihoney, many of his colleagues come to Dr. Simon to have small burns or scars treated, which the good-natured doctor readily cures with liquid Medihoney. "If the burn is grade two or less, Medihoney is very effective. If deeper, then you first need surgical debridement," Dr. Simon cautioned, adding, "Any complications must be handled under the supervision of a physician."

When asked about the future of wound care, Dr. Simon smiled warmly. "Patients will request Medihoney from doctors, because the evidence speaks for itself." While other honey varieties such as cornflower, thyme, lotus, and conifer have successfully been applied to wounds, the certification of Medihoney ensures the prescribing doctor a consistent product.

## NEWBORNS AND HONEY

Shortly after Mel's birth, Israeli doctor's opened up his tiny chest to perform corrective heart surgery.[12] His chest cavity swelled and the doctors could not close his sternum back up. The young boy struggled for life. By the twelfth day after his heart surgery, his open chest wound started to leak pus. The hospital staff took a swab and discovered *Pseudomonas aeruginosa*, a common bacteria in neonatal intensive care units, infected his wound.

To clear the infection, doctors hooked baby Mel up to an IV drip of antibiotics. The wound was treated with a topical application of sulfamylon and povidone-iodine. But the wound failed to respond, and Mel's chest cavity remained wide open.

As the little boy struggled for survival, the area between the lungs that houses the heart, esophagus and the lymph nodes—the mediastinum—swelled with inflammation. Doctors determined Mel had developed MRSA. Luckily the small boy remained stable despite 14 days of intensive medical care. His chest wound oozed thick pus infected with multiple organisms.

When Mel's conditioned still hadn't improved by the thirtieth day, doctors took him off antibiotics. His infected wound was cleaned with normal saline. Then the medical staff spread 5-10 ml of commercial, unprocessed, unpasteurized normal honey on his chest, replacing the dressing two times every day.

Six days of honey treatment and Mel's swelling finally subsided. Healthy new tissue replaced the necrotic. Swabs revealed the bacterial infections had disappeared. Two weeks after starting honey treatments, Mel's wound had completely closed.

When the doctors followed up a year later, Mel was in fine health and the skin remained healthy looking. Since Mel's successful results the Israeli doctors continue to use honey to treat non-responsive and infected surgical wound of neonates at the Chaim Sheba Medical Centre in Tel Hashomer.

If their young patients' wounds still ooze pus and their bacterial swabs remain positive after 14 days of topical treatments and systemic antibiotics, the team of doctors switches the patients to the honey dressings.

All nine of their young patients, who failed to respond to conventional treatment, showed signs of healing after five days of honey dressings. Some patients healed faster than others, but all were closed, clean and sterile within 21 days of starting the honey therapy. One patient healed in only five days, while the average across all nine patients was 12 days. None of the newborns showed had any negative reactions to the honey dressings, indicating that honey dressings can be used successfully on extremely young patients.

## WOUND INFECTIONS AFTER CESAREAN SECTIONS AND HYSTERECTOMIES

When a mother delivers a baby via cesarean section, doctors either make a vertical cut or a horizontal 'bikini' cut just above the public bone. After delivery the surgical wound is sutured. The surgical wound surgeons leave behind is prone to infection. Weakened from the ordeal, a woman develops fever. The inflamed wound becomes tender to the touch, pus forms and the wound bed deteriorates. Swabs taken from the wound confirm bacterial infection. Blood samples prove free of infection, indicating the bacteria remained localized to the wound bed.

To alleviate the suffering of his female patients, Dr. Noori S. Al-Waili of the Dubai Medical Center in the United Arab Emirates wanted to apply honey dressings. He procured pure Yemeni honey and tested its antibacterial activity against bacteria isolated from his patients' wounds. He took small discs of filter paper and soaked them in undiluted honey. Then he placed these circular scraps into nutrient rich agar plates seeded with the isolated bacteria. With plenty to eat, the bacteria normally multiply and rapidly cover the whole plate. But the honey-impregnated discs were surrounded by large empty circles - rings of inhibition where the bacteria simply could not grow. Dr. Al-Waili had confirmed his honey could halt the growth of the bacteria inhabiting his patients' wounds.

Fifty women fell under Dr. Al-Waili's care; 31 with infected cesarean sections and another 19 with abdominal hysterectomies. He randomly assigned half of his patients to receive twice daily applications of the active Yemeni honey, applied after the wound was rinsed with saline and then covered with gauze bandages.

The other patients received conventional antiseptics. Nurses washed the wounds with saline, then applied 70 percent ethanol and antimicrobial povidone-iodine, and finally dressed the wound with gauze.

Since this trial was conducted in 1999, when few trials had been completed with honey, both groups continued to receive systemic antibiotics to combat the specific types of bacteria infecting their wounds. Daily wound swabs allowed the medical team to track infection rates.

The women treated with honey responded immediately. After only four to five days of treatment, fever and local signs of inflammation disappeared in 14 of the 25 women. Wound swabs confirmed bacteria no longer

## Time to Healing

| Treatment | # of patients | Negative culture (days) | Healing (days) | Hospital stay (days) | Antibiotics used (days) | Scar size (mm) |
|---|---|---|---|---|---|---|
| Pure, active honey | 14 | 4.57 | 8.7 | 8.1 | 5.57 | 3.64 |
|  | 8 | 6.88 | 12.2 | 10.0 | 7.88 | 2.50 |
|  | 4 | 9.25 | 14.8 | 12.0 | 9.75 | 5.75 |
| 70% ethanol | 12 | 11.00 | 15.1 | 13.3 | 12.00 | 7.58 |
| & povidone- | 6 | 17.30 | 26.8 | 22.0 | 18.30 | 13.80 |
| iodine | 6 | 20.20 | 31.0 | 30.3 | 21.20 | 5.17* |

* Size of scar after resuturing

inhabited their wounds and the following day, Dr. Al-Waili discontinued systemic antibiotics. He removed the remaining surgical sutures and the wounds healed with minimal scars eight to ten days after commencing the honey dressings. The surgical wounds of another eight women cleared in seven days and the women were released from the hospital after ten days. Within two days of returning home the surgical wounds healed. The remaining four cleared in nine days. The recovering women were released from the hospital 12 days after commencing treatment and their wound finished healing three days later.

The topical ethanol and povidone-iodine treated wounds cleared and healed at a much slower rate. Twelve women took 15 days to heal, another six required 27 and the last six needed 31 days. Although all patients were on systemic antibiotics, their wounds only cleared after 11, 17 and 20 days. Sadly the surgical wounds of the final six women required resuturing; increasing their hospital stay to 30 days. (See table on left.)

Not only did the women treated with honey dressings heal faster and require shorter durations of antibiotics, they also had significantly smaller scars after their ordeal. At the time this study was conducted in 1999, few clinical trials testing honey's ability to clear wound infections had been completed. For ethical reasons Dr. Al-Waili felt it best to continue the use of systemic antibiotics until the wound cleared. Bacterial infections can migrate from surgical wounds into the blood stream and trigger septic shock, a life-threatening condition that causes a severe drop in blood pressure.

The women's large surgical wounds treated with honey healed well and not one required resuturing. Dr. Al-Waili concluded, "Honey application is inexpensive, safe and effective in (the) treatment of postoperative wound infection."[13]

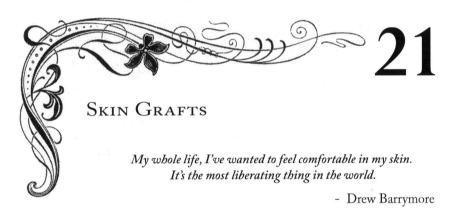

# 21

## Skin Grafts

*My whole life, I've wanted to feel comfortable in my skin.*
*It's the most liberating thing in the world.*

— Drew Barrymore

The Ayurvedic surgeon Sushruta invented skin grafts almost 3,000 years ago, as mentioned previously, earning him the honorary title as the father of plastic surgery. Despite his success other surgeons outside of the region failed to emulate the technique. During the next few thousand years only a few anecdotal reports of skin grafts occur.

In Bologna, Italy in 1597, Gaspare Tagliacozzi referenced skin transplants in his celebrated medical treatise, the first mention of such surgical skills in the Western world.[1] Another 200 years passed before Baronio Giuseppe of Milan reported a series of successful skin transplants executed on sheep.

One of the earliest Americans to specialize in plastic surgery, Jonathan Mason Warren was the third generation in his family to attend Harvard Medical School and earned his medical degree in 1832. He performed a nose reconstruction from a forehead skin graft in 1837, and developed a total skin graft procedure using a donor site from the arm in 1840. His contemporary, Joseph Pancoast, Professor of Surgery at Jefferson Medical College in Philadelphia, Pennsylvania, successfully reconstructed noses and earlobes by using skin grafts in 1844.[2]

Although skin grafting has been known for centuries, widespread interest only developed in the 19th century. Through the work of the two French surgeons Reverdin and Olliver, who rediscovered the art of skin grafting and improved upon it, the surgical process became more common.[3] Over the years numerous surgeons contributed to and refined the grafting technique.

Reconstructive surgeons typically apply split-thickness skin grafts to cover skin imperfections. The top layer of skin, the epidermis, has no blood vessels. Nutrients must diffuse into this top skin layer from the dermis below. A split-thickness skin graft transplants the entire epidermis and part of the underlying dermis from a donor site. The dermis contains glands and hair follicles lined with epithelial cells that can divide and generate a variety of different skin cells.

Split-thickness grafts are hardy, surviving despite imperfect conditions. Plastic surgeons use them to resurface large wounds. Because they don't contain the whole underlying dermis, they have greater fragility than full-thickness skin grafts. Once transplanted, the split-thickness skin graft often appears lighter or darker than surrounding tissue.

## DON'T FORGET THE DONOR SITE

Thighs make excellent donor sites. Once harvested, the donor site must regenerate new skin, a painful healing process that requires ongoing wound care. Much like in a second degree burn, common problems include infection, delayed healing, scar formation and pain. According to plastic and reconstructive surgeon Dr. Aykut Misirlioglu from the Lutfi Kirdar Kartal Education and Research Hospital in Istanbul, Turkey, "An ignored split-thickness skin graft donor site has often created a bigger problem for the surgeon than the original defect."[4] Patients also often complain of greater pain at the donor site.

To avoid complications, the optimal dressing should promote healing, reduce pain and inhibit infection. In chronic wound healing honey demonstrates all of these qualities. Common dressings include hydrocolloid and polyurethane films, which provide a moist wound healing environment to speed recovery. Unfortunately large wounds with high levels of fluid overwhelm the dressings in a few days and collect fluid underneath the dressing. This fluid must be drained off or the dressing replaced. Sometimes the dressings adhere to the wound bed, making them difficult and painful to remove.

Due to these drawbacks, Dr. Misirlioglu and his associates decided to compare the response of donor sites to hydrocolloid dressings and unprocessed, undiluted honey. Using an electrical dermatone, Dr. Misirlioglu harvested a two inch wide strip of skin no deeper than 0.014 inches from the patient's thigh.

For the first group of 42 patients, one half of the wound was treated with honey, while the other half received one of three different dressings: paraffin soaked gauze, hydrocolloid dressings or saline-soaked gauze.

A second group of 44 patients required two skin grafts, one from each thigh. Instead of splitting the treatment on a single wound, honey was applied to one leg and the other received one of the three alternative treatments.

Honey proved superior to both the paraffin and the saline soaked gauze dressings. Patients complained of less pain because the honey forms a thin, protective layer on the wound and prevents contact with the air. The team of surgeons found no significant differences in healing times between the honey dressings and the hydrocolloid dressings, although wound leakage occurred in 22 of the 29 hydrocolloid dressings. They concluded that honey could be a more cost-effective alternative to hydrocolloid dressings.

The Turkish team of surgeons never tested the antibacterial activity level of their honey, nor mentioned the floral source. Perhaps they would have seen higher rates of healing with a more active honey. Their results demonstrate honeys potential in healing skin graft donor sites and should encourage additional clinical trials.

## JEM'S STORY OF SURVIVAL: HONEY FOR SKIN LESIONS

Sprightly Jem's muscles ached and he felt nauseous on a Saturday evening in January, 1999.[5] "I got up a few times in the night to be sick and then I collapsed."[6] Panicked by the sudden onset of his illness, the family called an ambulance to take the sick 15- year-old to the hospital. "I remember being told that I had to go to (the) hospital and asking Mum to find my T-shirt, and I sort of remember thanking the ambulance driver for giving me a lift, but that's it."

Jem fell unconscious as his body fought against meningococcal septicemia, a lethal infection that had caused his blood pressure to plummet. The bacteria that cause meningococcal illnesses, a strain called *Neisseria meningitides,* live in the throat and back of the nose. One out of every five individuals carries them around without falling ill but they can cause meningitis. In Jem, the bacteria had punched through the protective mucosal lining of his throat and entered his bloodstream, where they rapidly reproduced and flooded his system with toxins, inducing septic shock.

Immediately upon Jem's admission to the hospital, the emergency team resuscitated the boy, hooked him up to a breathing apparatus and full support system in the intensive care unit. As the toxins coursed through his body, Jem's kidneys failed.

The toxins flowing through Jem's veins are 10 times more destructive to skin than other body parts. They set off a dangerous cascade in the immune system that hampered sufficient blood flow. Blood leaked out of his arteries and veins, and sporadic blood clots formed in small blood vessels throughout his body. His skin erupted in ugly lesions that bled. Gangrene set in and his extremities—fingers and feet—started to die off.

The team of doctors worked frantically to salvage his limbs, but both legs required amputation below the knee. "The surgeon told me straight out that I was going to have to have my legs amputated. That was one of the hardest things – basically watching my legs die before they could amputate." Jem also lost two fingers on each hand. He was lucky to survive. Twenty to 80 percent of people who contract fulminant meningococcal sepsis do not.

After two months of intensive care, the doctors transferred Jem to a regional burn and plastic surgery facility. The amputation sites where his fingers had been healed well, but his legs did not cooperate. To repair the damage the disease left behind, doctors transplanted skin from Jem's thighs and abdomen, but many failed to take.

"Then there was all the grafting—from the top of my legs and my stomach—and all the problems started. They tried everything to make the grafts work," Jem recalled. The donor sites proved troublesome too, causing Jem great pain whenever the nurses tried to change the dressings twice per week.

"I can't even begin to explain how painful it was just to have a small piece of dressing changed. The nurses tried everything to make it easier, like changing the dressings in the bath, but it was agony. And it got worse and worse. They gave me a mixture of nitrous oxide and oxygen, but towards the end that didn't work either. It felt like they were ripping my skin off."

The nurses tried a variety of dressings, including paraffin impregnated bandages, alginate and hydrocolloid dressings. Swabs of his lower legs revealed a multitude of bacteria had taken up residence, including *Pseudomonas spp*, *Staphylococcus aureus* and *Enterococcus spp*. The nurses applied silver sulfadiazine cream to halt the infection, but it proved useless.

The nurses realized how excruciating the dressing changes were for Jem. Frustrated and stumped for solutions, Jem's physicians called in a tissue viability team. Registered nurse Cheryl Dunford, who worked as a tissue viability specialist at Salisbury District Hospital in the UK at the time, was called in to advise on Jem's wound care. She implemented a multi-layer dressing to ease the pain and cleanse the wound. Although Jem's wounds initially responded favorably, the dressings had to be replaced too frequently, making them unsuitable.

None of the dressings worked right and Jem continued to suffer incredible pain during each dressing change. "We were at a loss," Cheryl Dunford explained.[7] Wound debris accumulated, putting Jem at greater risk of infection.

"I was walking along a corridor with one of the plastic surgeons, who was from India. He talked about how in India they used honey in wounds," Cheryl Dunford said. She had recently read an article by Dr. Rose Cooper on how honey eliminated the bacteria pseudomonas isolated from burn victims, one of the three culprits invading Jem's wound.

Although she hadn't read anything about honey's use for wound care, "I had one of those light bulb moments," she said. She made the connection between Cooper's article and Jem's struggle to heal.

"Oh, I wonder if it might work," she thought and decided to find out, so she wrote to Dr. Cooper, professor of microbiology at the Cardiff School of Health Sciences at the University of Wales. Dr. Cooper kindly mailed her some gamma irradiated absorbent dressing pads impregnated with 25-35g of active manuka honey.

After clearing the novel treatment method with the hospital, Cheryl Dunford applied the dressing to Jem's right leg. His other leg continued to receive conventional therapy, acting as a comparative control.

"It was obvious to me really quickly that the honey was doing the job," Jem said. "For a start it didn't stick as badly, but one of the main things I noticed was that the smell wasn't nearly as bad. I'm not saying that it was worse than the pain, because the pain was bad, but the smell was one of the things that bothered me most. As soon as we started using the honey, the smell improved."

The staff started treating all of his wounds with the manuka dressings. The odor dissipated after the first dressing change, which had a profound effect on Jem. "Wound odor has a very demoralizing effect on patients," Cheryl Dunford said. "Practitioners aren't always aware of this. They're so used to malodor, it doesn't really register."[8]

"Jem had had the traumatic experience of having to live with his decaying limbs and their smell before the decision was made to amputate them," Cheryl Dunford explained.[9] "The association between smell and emotion is well recognized ...By eliminating the smell, Jem did not have such a strong trigger for his anxiety and was able to gain further control of his situation."

Jem's leg responded to the honey dressing straight away. Within a few days, healthy granulation tissue appeared. Wound swabs revealed the *Pseudomonas spp* and *Enterococcus spp* had been eliminated.

Surprisingly the staph infection lingered on, but didn't interfere with Jem's healing. The pain of the dressing changes lessened and the nurses could finally stop the general anesthesia. Six weeks after switching over to the manuka dressings, Jem received his last successful skin graft. Within 10 weeks of commencing the manuka honey dressings every one of his lesions had healed completely with minimal scar tissue.

Shortly after his hospital discharge, Jem was fitted with prosthetic legs. "I've had my new legs for a few weeks, but I've been warned not to overdo it. I've got to build up gradually, but it's not going to take long. Within a few weeks I've gone from walking between parallel bars to running around on crutches."

Jem's remarkable recovery made international news headlines and he appeared on numerous television programs to discuss his experience.

The honey dressings used on Jem proved "highly successful and it took off from there", Cheryl Dunford said. She has traded her clinical work setting for a faculty teaching position in House Sciences at Southampton University in the United Kingdom. Many of her colleagues continue to utilize honey dressings, especially to eliminate bacterial infections. "Honey holds significant promise as an effective treatment in the management of wounds," she said.[10]

# *Interlude*

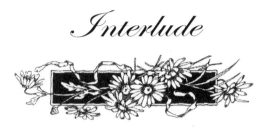

## *Honey for Burns*

SHOULD BE CONSTANTLY ON HAND READY FOR ANY EMERGENCY

About five years ago, it was my pleasure to have an old retired couple build a home beside me. They had been pioneer farmers first near Winona, Minnesota, and later in Saskatchewan. My wife and I very much enjoyed hearing their pioneering experiences, one of which follows:

In clearing the land of stumps in Minnesota, it was often necessary to bore holes in the larger ones and use blasting powder to split them. A farm hand, thinking the fuse had failed to ignite a charge, approached the stump and received a burning flash full in the face, which imbedded the grains of powder into the skin. No doctor was immediately available in those then remote parts, and the good mother made use of what she thought would bring the quickest relief. It was not known at the time whether the eyes were injured or not, but she lavishly smeared honey over the entire face and eyelids. A cloth mask was then fitted with only holes for the nose and mouth.

It was a matter of four or five days before a doctor examined the burns. He merely lifted the cloth and replaced it, saying, "you have used the best dressing that could be had". The result was that the entire face healed without a scar, the eyes were not injured and not one grain of powder remained. That he was not powder-marked for life was the most unusual thing.

Knowing this old couple (who have since passed to the life beyond) as I did, full credence may be given to this experience.

*Chas. E Phillips, St. Catharines, Ontario*
*Gleanings in Bee Culture, May 1933*

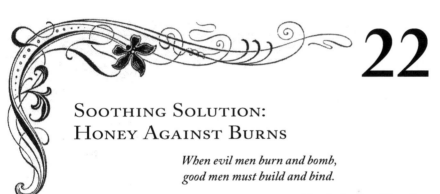

# 22

## Soothing Solution: Honey Against Burns

*When evil men burn and bomb,*
*good men must build and bind.*

- Martin Luther King, Jr.

*By* taming fire, we learned to light the darkness, burn fields to plant crops, protect ourselves against dangerous animals and drive away the chill of winter. As the children's story *Jungle Book* so vividly depicts, the power to harness fire gives humans the edge over the wilderness, permitting civilization to flourish.

Never to be completely tamed, nature still shows her unruly side: wildfires rage across vast stretches of land, unwatched candles ignite houses and natural and man-made explosions leave behind serious burns.

Burns are far too common. Fire and flames cause most injuries, with hot liquid scalds right behind.[1] Only car accidents claim more accidental loss of life. Every year 2.4 million Americans suffer burns.[2] Of these 650,000 burns are severe enough to warrant medical attention. Hospitals are inundated with 75,000 burn victims annually. Almost one third of those hospitalized are burnt over more than 25 percent of their body. Common victims include young children scalded by hot liquids.[3]

Despite advances in medical care, the successful healing of burns is still notoriously difficult to achieve. [4] After long bouts of hospitalization and rehabilitation, many are left disfigured and disabled. Prone to infection, burn wounds heal slowly. Survivors typically spend just over one day in the hospital for every percent of their total body surface area that is burnt - so a 30 percent burn typically requires just over a month's hospitalization.[5] In 2004 the cost to treat 32,500 burn victims topped $570 million dollars.[6]

Since our skin is the body's largest organ and the protective barrier that keeps out many infections, burns that destroy our defensive dermis can be deadly. The first description of burn victims and potential treatment can be found in the 54 foot long Ebers Papyrus, an ancient Egyptian document dating to approximately 1550 BC. It recommends bandaging burn wounds with honey as of the very first day.[7]

Keen observation plus trial and error must have guided Egyptian healers. As discussed in previous chapters, the antibacterial, anti-inflammatory and healing properties of honey soothe painful burns, clear infections and stimulate new tissue growth.

A recipe book compiled in the 17th and 18th centuries recounts how honey saved a lady from a terrible ordeal:

> At Rome a Lady had the misfortune to be severely burned almost all over her whole Body by her Cloathes taking fire. To give temporary ease to the Torture a Domestic had recourse to some Honey, which had so good an effect that in Nine Days she was perfectly cured by the use of this remedy alone.[8]

With the advent of modern medicine, we discarded volumes of knowledge on the medicinal benefits of nature's products. Only recently have we started to reexamine the therapeutic properties of natural products, spurred in part by the general public's desire for natural remedies.

Pharmaceutical companies have even sent agents into remote rainforests to speak with local medicine men about what plants they use to gain insight into potential new products.[9] After isolating the beneficial properties in the lab, pharmaceutical companies can apply for patents with large potential profits. Pharmaceutical products derived from biological resources were estimated to be worth $43 billion worldwide in 1995.[10]

Up until World War I, modern medicine knew little about caring for burn victims. Skin grafts along with large doses of pain medication then became routine. Before the 1950s burns on less than 50 percent of your body proved fatal half of the time. Currently 95 percent of all burn patients survive the ordeal.[11] Even some people that have burned over 95 percent of their body manage to survive, although they frequently have lingering physical impairments and psychiatric trauma.

Burn victims take time to heal. The costs of hospitalization and treatment are high. While the average hospital stay is just over five days, burn victims typically take almost nine days. The average cost for burn victim hospitalization runs $17,300 compared with $9,000 for all other types of hospitalization.[12]

Though improved treatments have significantly lowered the death rate since the early 20th century, burn victims are still almost twice as likely to die as other hospital patients. Every year burns claim 4,500 lives. Elderly patients have the most difficult time recovering from their burn wounds; over 15 percent of burn victims 65 years or older die during hospitalization.[13]

## DEGREES OF A BURN

Proper treatment of a burn depends on the severity and location of the wound. Burns are traditionally classified into three categories: first, second and third degree burns, depending on how deep the skin damage penetrates.

## FIRST DEGREE

Unlike murder, first degree burns are the least severe. They damage only the thin outer skin surface, the epidermis. The skin typically turns red and the burn casualty experiences minor pain at the burn site. Sunburns characteristically fall into this category. Sensitive to the touch, the skin takes on a reddish hue, which turns white when pressed. Burn centers now call such burns "superficial". The body replaces the entire upper skin layer every 45-75 days, so superficial burns cause no lasting scarring.

## SECOND DEGREE

Blisters mean the burn penetrated the dermis, the fleshy second layer of our skin directly beneath the epidermis. This is considered a second degree burn, also called a partial thickness burn. To protect the healing tissue underneath and deal with the damage the blisters fill with clear fluid; the body's mechanism for sending in repair troops.

Some hair follicles and sweat glands make their home deep in the dermis; deep partial thickness burns can hinder their performance. Nerve endings may also be damaged, resulting in reduced pain levels. Deep partial thickness burns often require skin grafts to heal.

## THIRD DEGREE

When a burn penetrates beneath the protective, fleshy cushion of our dermis to the subcutaneous fat and muscle tissue below, it's called a third-degree burn or full thickness burn. Third degree burns sever nerves, so the victim feels no pain at that site. However, surrounding tissues often sustain second degree burns, where nerve endings still receive signals the brain translates into pain.

The skin appears white, charred, brown or black and may be hard and leathery. Purplish fluid will frequently fill the burn area. Since the protective layers of skin have been destroyed, infections and complications are common. The tissue regions that make new skin cells have been destroyed. Third degree burns heal slowly, inflicting great pain. Tragically, such burns leave behind extensive scars, marking the survivor for life.

## PLAYING WITH FIRE

Men tinker around with fire more foolishly than women. According to the American Burn Association, 70 percent of all burn victims are men.[14] Most burn incidents occur in the home, most frequently from a fire or flame (42 percent) and scalds (31 percent).[15]

## TREATMENT OF SUPERFICIAL BURNS: FIRST DEGREE

Superficial burns heal themselves within three to five days. To ease the pain, rub on a soothing anti-inflammatory cream. Honey's anti-inflammatory properties render it the ideal remedy for light burns. Many simply smear straight honey onto the burn. Or combine it using the ancient Egyptian ratio of one part honey to two parts skin cream.

On a personal note, not too long ago I was pouring boiling water into a mug for tea. My husband started speaking to me and I looked over at him. Distracted I poured hot water over my hand. It cascaded down my knuckles before I realized what a silly thing I had done. My husband's warning shout brought me back to my senses.

Although most recommend placing a burn under cold water, I instead put a thick coat of honey on the back of my hand. It immediately stopped air flow to the burn and cut off the pain. The hand never blistered and the redness on the knuckles quickly disappeared.

In a clinical trial conducted in 1991 on 104 patients, an Indian burn surgeon compared the effects of pure, undiluted honey versus the most common burn treatment of silver sulfadiazine.[16] After one week 91 percent of the honey treated wounds were sterile, compared with a meager seven percent of the burns treated with silver sulfadiazine. After 15 days, 87 percent of the honey treated wounds had healed compared to 10 percent of the silver group. The doctors concluded that honey proved to be an ideal burn treatment, as it relieved pain and reduced scarring.

### TREATMENT OF PARTIAL THICKNESS BURNS: SECOND DEGREE

Partial thickness burns destroy part of the protective dermis, and so take longer to heal. Burns raze our defenses, leaving us susceptible to infections. To halt invading bacteria, burn victims often receive antibiotics.

To speed the healing process, wound care specialists typically remove the dead tissue through debridement. Large sections of necrotic tissue require surgical debridement, a painful procedure. Using a scalpel, scissors or sharp implement the yellow, tan or black tissue is physically scraped from the wound bed. The body can also self-generate and release enzymes to breakdown and digest dead tissue - a process known as autolytic debridement.

As mentioned previously, honey stimulates autolytic debridement.[17] In burns treated with honey, the dead tissue naturally detaches from the wound bed. The slough then lifts off easily with dressing changes, eliminating the need for surgical debridement. Doctors are still unsure how honey generates this greater activation of the body's natural repair system, but the continuous production of hydrogen peroxide may play a role.

The use of honey on partial thickness burns also reduces inflammation. Swelling tends to diminish and pain subsides. By decreasing the swelling, referred to as edema by medical doctors, blood can circulate more freely through the capillaries. The free flow of blood delivers oxygen to the affected tissue, stimulating tissue regeneration.

With a low pH, honey acidifies the wound site. This increases the release of oxygen from hemoglobin, the red blood cell protein responsible for transporting oxygen from the lungs to the rest of the body.[18] At the burn site, the cells put this oxygen to good use in tissue generation and wound repair.

Honey also contains antioxidants, which neutralize damaging free radicals. While free radicals can be beneficial in the earliest stage of wound healing as they have antibacterial properties, they later delay the generation of new tissue. This may be why partial thickness wounds sometimes develop into full thickness deep wounds that require skin grafting.

## TREATMENT OF FULL THICKNESS BURNS: THIRD DEGREE

Deep burns are the most challenging to treat. The cells that restore and heal the body have been wiped out and no longer exist. Doctors must transplant intact skin from healthy donor sites, grafting on a new dermis and epidermis; the top two layers of skin that can generate new cells.

Once the body accepts this new skin at the burn site, the transplant can generate additional tissue at the burn site. Enterprising surgeons in India have even kept skin grafts alive in pure solutions of honey at room temperature for five to 12 weeks.[19] When removed from storage, the grafts were firm and yellow-brown in color. To reconstitute the tissue, they were soaked in saline, which restored them to a normal texture and improved the color.[20] The honey stored grafts were then transplanted onto 20 burn patients. Five days later, the surgeon removed the dressing. Grafts stored less than six weeks had 100 percent acceptance rates, while those stored up to 12 weeks had an 80 percent acceptance rate. Two and three weeks after grafting the skin transplants adhered firmly, confirming the grafts had been accepted.

A medical trial demonstrated that while honey is highly effective in superficial and partial thickness burns, deep burns fare better with early tangential excision—a surgical procedure that removes successive layers of tissue from the wound—and skin grafts. These two surgical interventions reduced healing times and resulted in shorter hospital stays.[21]

The 25 deep burn patients who received honey treatment healed more slowly, but 14 of them never needed skin grafts. The surgeon never determined the antibacterial potency of the honey used in this trial. If the honey lacked high levels of glucose oxidase or non-peroxide activity, it would fail to eliminate the bacteria that frequently colonize deep burns and impede the healing process. An active honey quickly eliminates bacteria from the wound, assisting the body as it heals itself. Additional trials using an active honey for the treatment of deep burns are needed.

Animal trials that examined deep dermal burns on pigs[22,23,24] found that honey speeded the formation of new skin cells, improved healing times and reduced inflammation of the wound in comparison with silver sulfadiazine, sugar or no treatment. Since animals can't be swayed by the placebo effect, the trial results encourage further inquiry. Additional clinical trials to evaluate the benefits of honey for third degree burns would be useful.

## HONEY VS. SILVER DRESSINGS FOR SUPERFICIAL BURNS

Modern medicine in developed countries often implements skin grafts to treat second degree burns, a costly intervention. In developing countries like India, such advanced care is too expensive for most clinics.[25] Burn surgeons continually seek out inexpensive yet effective alternatives to prevent infection, decrease fluid loss and enhance new tissue growth in their patients.

In first and second degree burns, the remaining tissue still has the ability to regenerate skin cells to replace lost skin. Keeping infection at bay is the attending physician's primary concern. A moist wound environment promotes new skin formation and healing, but also spreads a welcome mat for bacteria to take up residence.

Honey's natural antibacterial properties make it an ideal dressing for burns. In an Indian clinical trial, a burn surgeon compared unprocessed, undiluted honey to silver sulfadiazine impregnated gauze.

Fifty patients with superficial thermal burns covering 10 to 40 percent of the body surface were treated within six hours of sustaining their injury. The burn surgeon took culture swabs to analyze their wound infections, and then washed the site with normal saline. For half the patients, he then applied 15-30 ml of pure honey directly onto the burn surface and covered it with sterile gauze. The other half received silver dressings. While the silver dressings were exchanged every day, the honey dressings were replaced every other day.

The surgeon noted wound progress every second day. Additional wound swabs were taken after one week and three weeks. By the end of the first week, only four patients in the honey group still had wound exudation; healthy granulation tissue had formed in the others. Eight of the patients receiving silver dressings still had wound exudation. Of the remaining 17 wounds, 15 had a hard, dry black necrotic eschar that the surgeon surgically removed so healthy granulation tissue could form.

By the third week, pus and slough could no longer be found in any of the honey treated wounds, while five silver dressing patients showed these signs of bacterial infection. All of the honey treated wounds healed by this time compared to 84 percent of the wounds treated with silver dressings. The remained 16 percent of unhealed wounds degraded from partial thickness to deep full thickness burns and required skin grafts.[26]

Additional clinical trials compared honey treatments in partial thickness burn to other conventional treatments such as OpSite*, a transparent waterproof film dressing.[27, 28, 29, 30] Honey consistently reduced the healing time, minimized scar tissue and sterilized a greater percentage of wounds than the conventional treatments. The smallest trial involved 64 burns, while the largest included 900 patients. Such widespread success should instill consumer confidence in using honey to treat partial thickness burns.

## Two Halves and Honey Makes Whole

Conventional treatments for burns include paraffin-impregnated gauze, gel-forming agents known as hydrocolloids, and polyurethane film or foam. To reduce the risk of infections, many burn care specialists treat singed flesh with creams containing silver. Silver functions as a broad spectrum antimicrobial, knocking back a wide range of microbes.

Since honey also has antimicrobial properties and has enjoyed wide success in eliminating bacteria from wounds, a team of physicians at the Burn Center POF Hospital of Wah Cantt, Pakistan decided to compare the effectiveness of honey and silver dressings in a clinical trial.[31] Patients often heal at very different rates. To eliminate such inherent differences in healing times, the doctors only enrolled 150 individuals with two burns of similar severity. One of the matched wounds was treated with honey, while the other received standard silver dressings.

The burns all occurred within 24 hours of commencing treatment. The burn sites included matched burns of both feet, legs, arms or hands, the left and right side of the abdomen, back or chest. None were greater than 40 percent of the total body surface area.

Immediately upon entering their care, the burn staff rinsed the patient's wound with water or normal saline solution. If the patient had burnt both their hands, a commercially available pure honey was applied to one hand and silver sulfadiazine cream to the other. Neither the patient nor the nurse were informed which side received a particular treatment, an effort to blind the patient and evaluator of wound progression. Every day the dressings for both treatments were replaced twice. After two weeks of treatment, clinical staff procured a wound swab to evaluate infection rates.

Pure, commercial honey treatments triggered more rapid healing. While the burns treated with silver sulfadiazine typically healed in 15.6 days, those receiving honey healed completely in 13.5 days. All the honey treated wounds healed within 21 days; the others took as long as 24 days.

Some burn wounds stubbornly refuse to heal regardless of the treatment, refusing to generate new tissue until new skin has been grafted onto the wound. The burn sites of eight patients in the honey treated group failed to heal. *Pseudomonas*—the most common burn wound infection—invaded six of those wounds and impeded recovery. In contrast, 29 wounds tested positive for bacterial infection in the silver sulfadiazine group and never healed. *Pseudomonas* populated 27 of those wounds, while *Escherichia coli* infected the other two. All of these patients received successful skin grafts.

### Healing Time of Burn Wounds

| Time to Heal | Honey (150) | SSD (150) |
|---|---|---|
| < 10 days | 30 | 13 |
| < 14 days | 92 | 67 |
| < 19 days | 18 | 10 |
| < 21 days | 2 | 21 |
| > 24 days | 0 | 10 |
| Mean healing time | 13.47 | 15.62 |

According to a survey conducted in 1998 honey is a widespread home remedy for burns and the preferred treatment of 5.5 percent of individuals worldwide.[32] However medical practitioners most commonly prescribe silver sulfadiazine dressings, an expensive option. The antimicrobial effect is the only benefit of silver sulfadiazine dressings, yet they can trigger devastating side effects including hepatic or renal toxicity; fancy medical terms for liver and kidney damage. In light of clinical trials that show improved healing with the use of honey compared to silver sulfadiazine dressings, perhaps doctors should reconsider their conventional approach to burns.

## Burn Wounds Prone to Infection

When burns destroy protective tissue, bacteria see the damaged defensive barrier as an opportunity to invade. The most common trespasser in burn wounds is *Pseudomonas aeruginosa*, a gram-negative bacteria that pervades soil and water. An opportunist, *P. aeruginosa* prefers moist habitats. It needs very little nutrients to survive, even setting up house in distilled water.

Immediately after being burnt the resulting wound is sterile. But the burn damage compromises the protective function of the skin. Shortly after the burn incident, bacteria multiply and proliferate on the wound surface, feeding on the necrotic tissue left behind.[33]

Frequently *P. aeruginosa* spreads to burn sites via touch. Improperly disinfected hands or surgical implements permit the bacteria to transfer from one individual to the next, where it quickly colonizes immunosuppressed patients. Burn management must attempt to sterilize the wound, so as not to impede the healing process.

As far back as 1951 doctors noted that when *P. aeruginosa* infected burns, it contributed to graft failure, delayed healing, systemic complications and patient death.[34] Antibiotics helped control the development of this bacterial invader, but over time the bacteria developed resistance to numerous drugs.

Scientists have isolated *P. aeruginosa* from the wounds of burn victims. They grow the bacteria, letting it multiply into large colonies on petri dishes. Honey is then added at different dilution rates to see how much is needed to kill the bacteria. On average an eight percent honey solution or less completely inhibits the growth of the bacteria.[35] So even when honey is severely diluted by discharged fluid from the burn wound, it will still stop the most common multi-resistant bacteria *P. aeruginosa* that loves to take up residence. Manuka honey causes *P. aeruginosa* cells to burst open and die. The few that survive are distorted in shape.[36]

## Pediatric Burns Respond Well to Honey

Dr. Bangroo, a pediatric surgeon from St. Stephen's Hospital in Delhi, India recently investigated the potential of honey compared to silver sulfadiazine dressings in speeding the recovery of his young patients.[37] Over a period of three years from January 2001 through December 2003, he treated 64 patients as young as six months with burns covering up to 50 percent of their total body surface. None were older than 12. Most of the young children's burns resulted from accidental scalding, a common danger for children below the age of five.[38]

Half of the patients were randomly assigned to honey dressings, while the other half received silver sulfadiazine on the burn surface. Twice a day, hospital staff bathed the young children with water and soap, sponged their bodies to gradually peel off the dead skin and then refreshed their wound dressings.

To track the cycle of bacterial infection, swabs were taken at the time of admission prior to any treatment, two days after treatment started and then every third day until the wound healed. Doctors determined the burn wounds of 49 patients were infected upon admission; 25 in the honey group and 24 in the silver sulfadiazine group. Among the resident bacteria were the notorious *Pseudomonas, Klebsiella, Staphylococcus aureus, Streptococci,* and *E. coli.* Interestingly only 14 of the 28 patients admitted within less than six hours of sustaining their wounds, and one of 15 patients who arrived within 12 hours, were free of infection. If the parents waited more than 12 hours before bringing their child in for treatment, bacteria had already moved in and taken up residence.

After one week of treatment, honey eliminated the bacterial infection in 23 of the 25 patients. Silver sulfadiazine only cleared three wounds; the other 21 remained infected. The honey sped up healing; healthy new tissue appeared within eight days compared to 14 days in the silver sulfadiazine group. Honey decreased swelling and the level of wound exudates. Black, hard, necrotic eschar—a common feature of burn wounds—never formed. The only drawback to the honey dressings was a stinging pain immediately after application, which subsided within the hour. Injection of pain relievers eliminated this side effect.

Dr. Bangroo's study clearly demonstrated honey dressings effectively treat burns in very young patients. Honey creates a physical barrier on the burn surface and nourishes the repair troupes fighting to rebuild the damaged tissue, promoting the growth of healthy new skin. "These properties of honey make it an ideal and cost-effective dressing for burn patients,"[39] he noted.

## Military Major Mitigates Burns

As the former capital of a princely state, the city of Bahawalpur, Pakistan enjoys the prestige of many famous palaces. The city, the twelfth largest in Pakistan, is home to a Combined Military Hospital staffed by Pakistan's Army Medical Corp., a prestigious group of doctors.

Local residents frequent the busy outpatient clinics of the hospital, seeking help for a wide variety of ailments. From September 2002 until August 2003, Major Dr. Asher Ahmed Mashhood treated 50 patients for first and second degree burns.[40] As industrial burns decreased in frequency, he noted young children and housewives now made up the majority of burn victims. Often poor, they need inexpensive wound care solutions. This region of the world has a long tradition of healing with honey. Both Ayurvedic masters Sushruta and Chakra applied honey for wound care. Burns received a honey paste under Sushruta's healing touch.[41]

In light of honey's long use in wound care, the Major decided to compare pure, unprocessed honey to the standard burn ointment silver sulfadiazine. According to Major Dr. Mashhood burn doctors face the formidable task of alleviating pain and preventing complications in agonizing burn wounds. In well-equipped burn facilities such care is easy to provide and the outcomes are typically very good. But in many parts of the world, doctors confront serious injuries armed with only the most basic supplies.

In regions of widespread poverty, the cost of treatment forms a major hurdle to the proper care of burns. Patients simply can't afford expensive treatments. Cheap and readily available, honey makes an attractive alternative.

The 50 burn patients treated by Major Dr. Mashhood and his staff were equally divided. All wounds were cleaned with normal saline, then half received daily applications of a thin layer of pure, unprocessed honey, while the other half were similarly dressed with one percent silver sulfadiazine cream. Over 50 percent of the honey treated burns healed within two weeks and the rest healed within four. The burns treated with silver sulfadiazine didn't fare quite so well; only 20 percent healed within two weeks, 60 percent by four weeks and all completed the healing process after six weeks.

The honey treatments substantially reduced the pain felt by patients. Pain completely subsided in more than one third of honey treated patients by the end of the first week. Eighty percent stated the pain disappeared after two weeks, while all 25 patients were free of pain by the third week. Silver sulfadiazine treatments eliminated pain in 16 percent of patients by the end of the first week, 44 percent after two weeks, 72 percent by the third week and all 25 patients after four weeks of daily dressing changes.

Patients preferred the honey dressings, which could easily be cleansed with saline during dressing changes. In contrast, the silver sulfadiazine cream formed a thick layer over the wound. Wound care staff removed this via rubbing and patients often required general anesthesia to counter the pain.

The main goal of using silver dressings is to stop bacterial infections. Yet the honey dressings cleared all the wounds within three weeks compared to five weeks for the silver dressings. The antibacterial activity of this honey was never tested and may have been quite low. A highly active honey may have cleared the wound infections even sooner.

Cost of care is an important factor in developing countries. A single honey dressing cost 1/10th the price of the silver dressing. Since the honey treated wounds healed substantially faster, fewer dressing changes are needed, further reducing the total cost of treatment.

While cost alone usually won't rule out potential treatments in developed countries, all nations seek to cut the cost of medical care. Honey is not only more cost effective, it speeds the recovery process compared to silver dressings, suggesting more healthcare professionals should consider adopting honey for burn therapy.

## HIDDEN BENEATH THE SILVER LINING

In the last decade, a plethora of expensive silver dressings has popped up on the market. For approximately 40 years, doctors have known silver functions as a broad spectrum antimicrobial, knocking back a wide range of microbes. Despite their high cost, silver sulfadiazine dressings (SSD) are the preferred treatment in chronic wounds and severe burn management.[42]

According to a plastic surgeon for burns, "Although it has been the preferred topical treatment, in practice SSD cream causes a moist uneven macerated eschar that is loose at the edges, thus promoting bacterial proliferation. Moreover, the eschar is difficult to shave off. As a result, SSD does not consistently prevent or suppress bacterial growth in large wounds."[43]

Chronic wounds and second or third degree burns heal slowly, so the wound bed frequently maintains contact with the silver dressing for four weeks or longer. Intact skin absorbs no measurable amounts of metallic silver, and so causes no increase of the metal in the blood stream.[44] Under normal circumstances, the body, its organs and tissues contain very low levels of silver - normal blood concentrations stay below 2.3 µg/l.[45]

Open wounds, in contrast, provide the silver access to the blood stream. Trials using silver tagged with radioactive labels demonstrated the metal accumulated superficially within two to eight hours after a single use. It took 28 days before the body fully expelled the metal again. The body cleared itself within four weeks, indicating a low absorption rate from a solo application. But silver dressings are now used for greater durations up to and exceeding four weeks. Such constant exposure increases the opportunity for negative effects on the body.

A burn patient treated with silver sulfadiazine (SSD) cream died from acute kidney failure after eight days of treatment. An autopsy uncovered an abnormally high silver concentration, 280 times that of a normal person.[46] Six hours after a burn victim's wounds were treated with a SSD cream, the silver level in his blood jumped as high as 50 µg/l - over 20 times the normal range of 2.3 µg/l.[47]

---

**Expensive Silver Dressings**

The United Kingdom's National Health Service spent about £100 million on wound care prescriptions in 2006-2007. Less than 15 percent of the prescriptions were for silver dressings, but cost the healthcare system £25 million.

At such high cost, one would expect the silver dressings promoted better wound healing. But two systematic reviews of clinical wound care trials failed to show any benefit to these expensive dressings.

Cited in National Prescribing Centre 2008

---

We simply do not know enough about the long term effects of such elevated silver levels. Clinical trials examining the detriments of long term exposure to silver dressings have not been completed.

Instead of alleviating the symptoms of burns, silver sulfadiazine treatments may actually increase a patient's risk of acquiring several detrimental health conditions. This includes neutropenia,[48] a life-threatening condition where the body lacks crucial defensive white blood cells that fight infection; an extremely dangerous situation for a burn victim. As previously explained, loss of protective skin—the body's largest defensive organ—leaves burn victims highly susceptible to infections.

The absorption of other metals such as lead has highly detrimental effects. Until further information is uncovered, perhaps we should err on the side of caution when applying ingredients the body can not quickly assimilate and process, especially in burn victims that require long periods of wound care. Long term treatments compound the problem of absorption. Honey contains only trace minerals in amounts the body can easily assimilate.

As recounted above, honey proved superior to silver sulfadiazine dressings in several randomized clinical trials.[49,50,51,52,53] Within one week, honey rendered burn wounds sterile in 91 percent of superficial burns, an additional trial demonstrated. Although silver dressings are supposed to be antibacterial, only seven percent of patients treated with silver sulfadiazine had sterile burns. In addition to eliminating bacterial infections that impede healing, the honey reduced scarring and relieved pain.[54] According to the supervising surgeon, "Relief of pain, a lower incidence of hypertrophic scar and post burn contracture (common complications of burns), low cost and easy availability make honey an ideal dressing in the treatment of burns."[55]

These clinical trials prove honey more effective than silver dressings, without the additional risk of potentially damaging systemic silver absorption. Further large scale trials would help confirm the benefits of honey in the management of burn wounds, where creating a sterile environment is the key to successful healing.

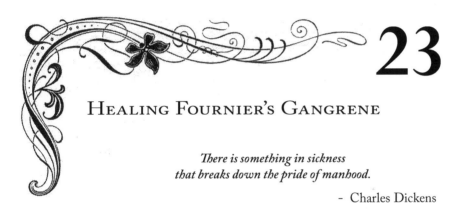

# 23

## HEALING FOURNIER'S GANGRENE

*There is something in sickness
that breaks down the pride of manhood.*

– Charles Dickens

$\mathcal{B}$orn in 1832, Jean Alfred Fournier, a French dermatologist and director of the Parisian hospital, Hôpital Saint-Louis,[1] dedicated himself to the study of sexually transmitted diseases during his lifetime. Fournier was taken aback when five healthy young men were assailed by a vicious and sudden onset of gangrene of their penis and scrotum. A bacterial infection promptly mushroomed from localized red swelling into rapid tissue death, what doctors call necrosis. If not reined in quickly, the spreading bacterial infection induces toxic shock, known as sepsis, and organs start to fail.

Ever since his early description in the French journal *Medecin Pratique* (Practical Medicine) in 1883, the disease has carried the French doctor's name. But it has claimed lives long before then. The diabetic King

Herod the Great of Judaea is suspected to have been afflicted with it.[2] In his report, Fournier noted the disease included 1) sudden onset in hitherto healthy young men, 2) rapid progression to gangrene and 3) absence of a definite cause.[3] Although he couldn't name a cause, he doubted sexual intercourse played a role as otherwise "we would see a great deal of the problem in our clinics".[4]

The picture of this debilitating disease shifted over the years. Although first described in healthy, young men, it most commonly strikes men in their fifties suffering from chronic alcoholism or diabetes. Individuals undergoing chemo or transplant recipients, who take meds to suppress their immune system, are also at increased risk. Swift and horrendous, this disease ravages the genitals and anus; it can strike women and young children, though male victims outnumber female 10 to one.[5]

While Fournier could find no definitive cause for the illness's rapid inception, doctors now know that it starts with inflammation near a site where bacteria find entry under the protective skin, most commonly coupled with an impaired immune system. Symptoms appear two to seven days after the initial breach. Doctors may require a meticulous investigation to locate the infection's portal of entry. Typically the bacteria breach the body's defense system via the urinary tract, the anus or through a tear in the skin.[6]

A troupe of about four bacteria—usually benign inhabitants of the gastrointestinal tract—interact synergistically to set off a violent cascade of events. Playing off one another, one bacterium produces a nutrient to feed another, which in response releases a toxin. The toxin protects both organisms from the individual's internal clean-up crew, so they avoid destruction.[7] Another organism produces enzymes that clot the blood vessels nourishing the region. The tissue becomes deprived of oxygen, which improves the growth of other bacteria. These microorganisms then release additional enzymes that digest the fascial barriers; the bacteria breach the body's deep fascial planes, connective tissues that wrap around large arteries and spread to sterile body regions previously off limits.[8]

Without oxygen, the overlying skin dies off. The bacteria feed on the dying flesh, releasing harmful toxins that further break down tissues and produce a repulsive stench. The wounds often leak pus resembling "dirty dishwasher fluid" and give off an "overwhelmingly repulsive odor".[9]

Some of the afflicted die within hours of the onset of physical symptoms, usually from toxic shock, uncontrolled bleeding when blood fails to clot, kidney or multiple organ failure. Doctors treating patients for

Fournier's gangrene have lost up to 80 percent of the individuals.[10] A review of 1726 cases found an overall mortality rate of 16 percent.[11]

Early symptoms include intense genital pain and a swollen scrotum, frequently accompanied by fever. Doctors habitually misdiagnose during the early stages, because the skin shows few signs of the disease. Once gangrene sets in, the patient's pain subsides as nerves die off. As the bacterial infection floods the body, delirium often escorts the toxic shock. Organs start to fail despite early recognition and aggressive management of the disease.

Because Fournier's gangrene degenerates rapidly, treatment is urgent. To slow down the bacterial rampage, doctors pump a cocktail of antibiotics into the patient. When tissues start to die off, the surgeon must promptly cut away any unhealthy skin. If the patient survives, such aggressive techniques typically require reconstructive surgery.

In a review on the management of Fournier's gangrene, the author writes:

> *More recently, the value of topical unprocessed honey has also been recognized and used, with an impressive acceleration of healing. Honey has a low pH of 3.6 and contains enzymes which digest dead and necrotic tissue. It contains antimicrobial agents to which the infecting organisms are usually sensitive. It also stimulates growth and multiplication of epithelial* (skin) *cells at the wound edges. These changes occur within a week of applying honey to the wound.[12]*

From April 2001 through May 2003, Dr. Subrahmanyam and Dr. Ugane from the Government Medical College Miraj and the General Hospital in Sangli, India treated 30 men with Fournier's gangrene. The surgeons obtained a varietal honey the bees made by foraging predominantly on the fragrant white flowers of *Syszygium cumini*, what the locals call Jamun - a tall tropical evergreen tree in the Myrtle family. Bacterial tests confirmed the honey was free of microorganisms.

Pieces of gauze were dipped in the honey and applied to the wounds of 14 men. The other 16 received similar gauze strips dipped in Edinburgh University Solution of Lime (EUSOL). EUSOL, an antiseptic solution of chlorinated lime and boric acid[13] was developed as a cheap and effective remedy for treating war wounds.[14] It's known for its ability to debride and control odor. The doctors then layered absorbent cotton pads over both treatments, finishing off with a final bandage. Staff refreshed the dressings daily.

The dead mass of yellow-gray soft tissue—what doctors call slough—disappeared from the wounds after one week in over half of the men treated with honey and in the rest by the end of the second week. The foul odor emanating from the festering genitals diminished after only two days, along with the inflammatory swelling.

Despite care, one man died among the men treated with honey, while two deaths occurred in the control group treated with EUSOL. Interestingly the honey treated men spent significantly less time in the hospital, returning home after an average of 28 day, while the EUSOL group spent four extra days under hospital care.

## Fournier's Gangrene in Nigeria

Another surgeon in Nigeria, Dr. Spencer Efem from the University Department of Surgery at the University Teaching Hospital of Calabar, used honey to treat Fournier's gangrene very successfully in 20 males, ranging in age from one month to 80 years. Inflicted individuals conventionally receive large doses of antibiotics, aggressive surgical debridement of necrotic tissue and adequate drainage.

"All surgeons agree," Dr. Efem states, "that this condition requires active and immediate surgical treatment by incision and drainage and wide excision of all necrotic and gangrenous tissues as the treatment of choice."[15] Yet his findings after treating 20 patients with honey call into question the validity of this standard approach.

Dr. Efem cleaned the wounds with normal saline and then applied 15 to 30 ml of pure, unprocessed honey directly onto each ulcer. Ten men had their large, festering wounds packed with honey soaked gauze. Dr. Efem then dressed the wounds with sterile gauze, before bandaging. Nineteen of the 20 men required no surgical intervention, while the final individual necessitated a round of suturing. All of the patients continued to receive a cocktail of antibiotics against the multitude of bacterial infections.

Within one week of commencing the honey therapy, wound odor dissipated, the swelling decreased and pus disappeared. The necrotic tissue separated naturally, lifting off without surgical intervention. Healthy, new skin appeared at the wound edges. The skin regenerated rapidly along the scrotum, leaving minimal or no scars behind. The only man who required surgical suturing had lost almost all of the skin on his scrotum to gangrene. Originally Dr. Efem had believed he would need to reconstruct the scrotum using skin grafted from the man's thigh. But in the end, the honey "produced such a remarkable regeneration of scrotal skin that reconstruction ...was abandoned in favor of secondary wound suturing."[16]

To see if honey proved more effective than the orthodox methods applied at that time in his hospital, Dr. Efem compared the results of his patients with 21 similar cases of Fournier's gangrene treated by other surgeons during the same time period. In all of these men, the doctors surgically debrided the gangrene, cutting away the rotting and dead tissues. The wounds failed to close in 19 individuals and required a second operation for re-suturing. Doctors harvested skin flaps from the thighs of two conventionally treated men to reconstruct their scrotums. Despite the aggressive care, three of the men died.

The traditionally treated men spent less time in the hospital and were released on average after four weeks, while those receiving honey spent four and a half weeks under Dr. Efem's care. But none of the honey group died, nor did they require reconstruction, nor two rounds of surgical intervention.

"The action of unprocessed honey on Fournier's gangrene is simply remarkable," Dr. Efem said. "When it is applied on the ulcer, it immediately halts the advancing necrosis. It debrides, sterilizes, deodorizes, and dehydrates the wound, and it stimulates actual regeneration of scrotal skin by rapid epithelialization. All these changes can be observed within 1 week of topical application."[17]

Honey's phenomenal results against this notoriously problematic disease should make it the remedy of choice, Efem believes.

## ALCOHOLICS AND DIABETICS

A team of medical doctors from the Department of Urology at the Hospital General de Zonano in Nuevo Leon, Mexico and the Indiana University Medical Center in Indianapolis, Indiana treated 38 patients with Fournier's gangrene.[18] To halt the progression of the debilitating disease, the team aggressively cut away all dead tissue along with any questionable flesh.

After aggressive surgical debridement, the doctors applied unprocessed honey to the ulcerated flesh. The honey treatment accelerated wound recovery so that by the tenth day the medical team saw signs of rapid healing and regeneration of lost skin.

The men afflicted with Fournier's gangrene ranged from 33 to 86 years-old with an average of 54. All lacked good personal hygiene and were from a low socioeconomic class. Two thirds had a long history of alcohol abuse. A drinking problem is a common thread in many who come down with Fournier's gangrene, as is diabetes. Diabetes inflicted two thirds of the men.

Before acquiring Fournier's gangrene, five of the men required surgery in the genital region. Such invasive procedures can provide bacteria with a point of entry, especially in immunosuppressed individuals.

The bacterial infection overwhelmed the immune response in one of the men and caused toxic shock. Despite broad-spectrum antibiotics and aggressive medical support, his system failed to recover from the onslaught and he died six days after the surgeons had surgically removed the dead genital tissue.

Honey is so effective in the treatment of Fournier's gangrene because it naturally debrides the wound, creates an antibacterial environment and locally generates oxygen that speeds the healing process. According to the team of doctors:

> *The action of unprocessed honey in Fournier's gangrene is effective, when it is applied on the ulcer, since it immediately halts the advancing necrosis, debrides, sterilizes, deodorizes, and absorbs fluid from the wound. Unprocessed honey also stimulates the regeneration of scrotal skin by rapid epithelialization by improving the tissue oxygenation and hence wound healing. All these changes can be observed within 1 week of topical application of honey.*[19]

Honey houses enzymes that digest dead and necrotic tissues. They play an important role in naturally debriding and cleaning dirty wounds. The continuous production of hydrogen peroxide from the enzyme glucose oxidase generates part of honey's antibacterial potency. By halting the bacterial infection colonizing the genitals in Fournier's gangrene, honey speeds recovery. The doctors found that unprocessed honey enhances the growth and multiplication of new skin cells at the edges of the wound, alleviating the need to perform reconstructive plastic surgery of the scrotum. While individuals afflicted with Fournier's gangrene typically require hospital stays of 40-120 days, the surgical team discharged their patients after an average of only 17 days. Honey undoubtedly played a significant role in the men's rapid recovery from such a debilitating disease.

The team of surgeons concluded, "Although uncommon in the Western world, Fournier's gangrene is a common cause of acute scrotal pain in developing countries. It is important to recognize the disease early and begin aggressive medical and surgical therapy. We recommend the use of unprocessed honey in those gangrenous wounds applied topically, and ... skin grafts ...where needed."[20]

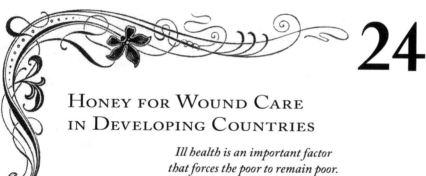

# 24

## Honey for Wound Care in Developing Countries

*Ill health is an important factor
that forces the poor to remain poor.
If they make a little bit of money,
one episode of illness can wipe them out.*

- Zafrullah Chowdhury,
Bangladeshi Public Health Advocate

*In* developed countries, patients frequently receive the latest medical treatment options. The cost of treatment is often a secondary concern. Developing countries feel pressure to catch up to the healthcare options offered in more developed countries, even at prohibitive costs.

"In the developing world (there is) a reluctance to stay with simple and still effective methods," Dr. Ronald Ingle from the Department of Family Medicine at the University of Limpopo in South Africa noted.[1] Yet doctors in developing countries often have limited budgets and must rein in costs, allowing them to care for more patients. If doctors can show that the simple remedies are as effective as the costly alternatives, it relieves some of the pressure from the endless tug of war between expensive medical advances and curtailing costs. Even in developed countries discussions over the cost of healthcare rage. Uninsured individuals who must pay for their own care up front benefit from cheap and effective remedies.

As part of Krijn Polinder's dissertation research in family medicine at the Medical University of Southern Africa, he studied the healing response of injured mine workers from two different mining operations. The 82 mine workers with shallow wounds or abrasions were randomly assigned to either receive topical applications of an unpasteurized, finely crystallized aloe honey or IntraSite Gel, a hydrogel wound care product consisting of 20 percent propylene glycol, two percent starch copolymer and 78 percent water.

All wounds were cleaned once daily with normal saline. Aloe honey was then applied from the 500 gram jar with individually wrapped wooden spatulas. The IntraSite gel comes in a sterile packet with a tearable opening and was squeezed directly onto the wound. For both treatments the amount applied depended on the wound's size but was enough to cover the entire site. To keep the wound treatment in place, Polinder covered it with OpSite; a transparent, adhesive film.

Both the aloe honey and the hydrogel treatments performed equally well. There were no statistical or clinical differences in rates of healing. However, honey was a substantially cheaper alternative costing four percent of the hydrogel product. "Honey is a safe, satisfying and effective healing agent," Dr. Ingle confirmed. "That it was comparably effective in the study allows the important conclusion that, in a natural form, honey is extremely cost-effective."[2]

### Cost Comparison of Honey and IntraSite Gel

|  | Average used per patient (g) | Purchase price (cost*/g) | Cost per gram* | Average cost* per patient |
|---|---|---|---|---|
| Honey | 35.17 | 7.00/500 | 0.014 | 0.49 |
| IntraSite Gel | 27.83 | 6.50/15 | 0.433 | 12.06 |

* Prices given in South African Rands

# Interlude

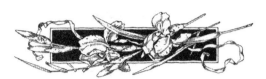

## Embalming the Dead

Instead of using honey during the mummification process, a mixture of beeswax and propolis—a sticky resinous substance bees gather from tree buds—helped embalm Egyptian pharaohs. While Egyptians did not usually preserve their dead in honey, other cultures such as the Babylonians buried their dead in honey to avoid the ravages of decay.[1]

According to a translation of an Ethiopic manuscript housed in the British Museum, Alexander the Great decried on his death-bed his body should be buried in honey:

> Then Alexander the king, the son of Ammon and the son of Olympias, commanded Chronos, the prince of blacksmiths, to make a leaden coffin, and to fill it with honey, and myrrh, and rose water, and he said, "Lay ye my body therein that it may be kept from corruption," and thus saying he gave up the ghost.[2]

Other authors recorded Alexander the Great's death with a slight twist:

> Philemon, the captain of his hosts, prepared his body for burial, and he anointed it with aloes, and placed it in a golden coffin, and poured over it the honey of the bees. Then he lifted it up and took it with him, and marched by day and by night to the city of Alexandria, and he brought forth the coffin and set it down among the people.[3]

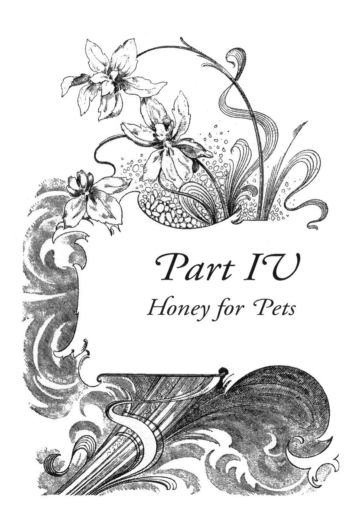

# Part IV

## Honey for Pets

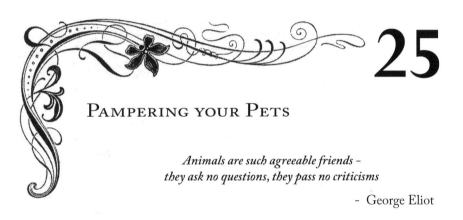

# 25

## PAMPERING YOUR PETS

*Animals are such agreeable friends –*
*they ask no questions, they pass no criticisms*

- George Eliot

Animals have kept us company since our earliest days; darling pets reward us with unconditional love and loyalty, farm animals provide nourishment and wild animals, though undomesticated, sometimes need a touch of care to survive. Honey can benefit many in the animal kingdom.

Just like us, animals suffer a variety of wounds and ailments, which can easily be treated with honey. As the word spreads about the beneficial properties of honey, more animals receive this super wound dressing. Most of the evidence of health benefits for animals remains anecdotal, although clinical trials have demonstrated the healing benefits of honey on pigs, mice and rats.

## Pet Hot Spots

Michael Liss, a homeopathic consultant and certified naturopathic doctor in Frederick County, MD recommends honey to treat pets, especially dogs who suffer from a painful condition called hot spots. "Honey is very effective against hot spots, because of its anti-inflammatory properties."[1]

Hot spots are localized areas of skin inflammation where bacterial infections often take up residence. Animals tend to bite, lick and scratch the region, worsening the hot spot. The area turns red and may ooze pus. Pets commonly lose hair in the infected region. The hot spots can grow rapidly in size, as the animal relentlessly scratches or chews at the irritated area. Dogs with thick coats are especially prone to this type of infection. As described in Chapter 3, active honey quickly eliminates bacterial infections. The anti-inflammatory properties soothe the itchiness, so your pet stops perturbing the area. You may need to use a conical collar on your pet for the first few days so they don't chew at the honey dressing.

## Call of the Wild

After a vicious shark attack left a giant, gaping wound on a young female sea lion, rescue staff decided to treat the large open wound with honey. "Sea lions are notoriously good at removing bandages and the necessary restraint for repeated bandage changes is stressful to the animal. She was not stable enough to undergo anesthesia, so whatever treatment was selected would need to be rapidly applied and minimally painful to an awake animal."[2] The sea lion received new honey applications every other day for 2 ½ weeks. Since honey naturally debrides a wound, the sea lions caregivers didn't need to perform painful surgical debridement. "The changes in the health of the wound were noticeable after the first bandage change." After two weeks, the sea lion joined other animals in an in-ground pool. Less than three months after her arrival at the care center she was released with only a small crescent shaped wound still visible.

## Dog Gone Allergies

Beekeeper and companion dog trainer Michele Crouse[3] regularly feeds honey from her hives to her four-year-old Staffordshire terrier named Bonnie to keep allergies at bay. "Bonnie has always had a hard time with allergies," Crouse says. "Her symptoms used to be worst in the spring and early summer, but they continued through the fall ragweed season. She rubbed her face, licked herself, especially on her feet and the inside of her thighs, and scratched on her stomach like crazy, creating dime-sized sores. She itched so much that the vet prescribed Benadryl and prednisone."

Instead of relying on over the counter medications, Crouse fed Bonnie a tablespoon of raw honey strained through a single filter twice per day. This daily regimen kept the four-legged Bonnie symptom free. "But if I forget for a week or so, the symptoms come right back. I know several other dogs, who have had the same response. They react to seasonal allergens until their owners put them on honey, and then they're fine."

## Going to the Dogs

The National Honey Board, which provides free recipes and consumer information (www.honey.com), wanted to see if honey might help our four-legged friends. They approached two non-profit pet shelters to see what effect honey would have when used with regular shampoos.[4] The 185 canine inhabitants at Denver's MaxFund and Georgetown's Clear Creek County Animal Rescue League were pampered like Hollywood stars, their fur massaged with honey during their next bath. The result: luxuriously clean and easy to comb coats, which thrilled the handlers.

Some of the volunteers at the shelters were professional groomers and 70 percent of the volunteers noted the honey bath left the pooches' coats feeling much softer. The honey made a winning impression; 72 percent of the volunteers who applied nature's first sweetener said they would use it in future grooming. An additional 10 percent said they would grab a bottle of honey if they had it on hand at home. Going to the dogs never sounded so good!

To try this remedy at home, simply work honey into the animal's coat at the same time you shampoo your pet, using equal amounts of each. The shampoo ensures the honey does not stick to the coat. Rinse off normally. Enjoy the radiant, healthy shine, effortlessly running your hands through that sumptuous coat.

## Weaning Pups

Sometimes a bitch doesn't produce enough milk for all of her pups. To help increase lactation certified homotoxicologist Marina Zacharias feeds the mother raw honey. With 18 years of experience, Marina is an expert in the natural rearing of dogs (naturalrearing.com).

"Honey is excellent at increasing lactation," she explains.[5] When you have to supplement the mother's milk and bottle feed pups, the holistic practitioner recommends the following weaning formula: 1 cup of goat's milk sweetened with 1 teaspoon of honey. Add two drops of sunflower oil for fat and dilute with 1 tablespoon pure water. This recipe helps the pups build up quickly. Raw honey works on dogs the same way it does on people."

She recommends therapeutic doses of one teaspoon of honey for a 60-70 lbs dog. When asked about the potential detrimental effects of sugar on dogs, she quickly pointed out that most dog food is loaded with hidden sugars, especially the moist ones. Treats also pack a lot of sugar. With trace minerals, antioxidants and antibacterial properties honey makes for a much healthier treat.

## DAIRY DELIGHT

Dairy cows often suffer from mastitis, a painful condition that causes inflammation of the udder. Typical symptoms include swelling, heat, redness and pain. The infection severely curtails milk production.

Most mastitis is caused by bacterial infections of *Staphylococcus*, *Streptococcus*, or *E. coli*, all of which cause inflammation of the teats and makes it difficult for the animal to pass milk. In an attempt to fight the infection, the dairy animal produces large quantities of white blood cells called leukocytes. These and other proteins create clots and flakes in the milk. The fat content also shrinks dramatically.[6]

Dairies treat this type of infection by injecting antibiotics into the teat canal. While the animal receives antibiotic medication, it must be pulled from dairy production lines. These drugs are fat soluble, which means they stay behind in the tissues for several days. The antibiotics must first clear the animal's system, before the cow can be used for milk production again. Otherwise traces of antibiotics contaminate the milk.

In lab experiments, honey successfully eliminates the bacteria which commonly cause mastitis.[7] Organic dairy facilities, which may not use antibiotics, could try applying active honey to infected teats. Unlike antibiotics, water soluble honey should not be retained in the tissues. Since the honey is not systemically absorbed, milk could be harvested from healthy teats immediately. Treated animals need only be withheld from milk production until the leukocyte levels return to normal. Honey could also be used to treat mastitis in other dairy animals such as sheep and goats.

In a clinical trial honey mixed into a cream made with bee pollen successfully reduced teat lesions in dairy cattle.[8] Small, two gram dollops of cream were gently massaged into sore and chapped teats after milking.

After one week, the cracked fissures and pseudo-cowpox lesions all but disappeared, leaving behind much smoother skin. The dairymen reported softer texture to the skin and greater ease of milking.

# References

PART I

## Two Million Blossoms

1. Swithers, S.E., and Davidson, T.L. (2008). A role for sweet taste: calorie predictive relations in energy regulation by rats. Behav Neurosci *122*, 161-173.

2. Fowler, S.P., Williams, K., Resendez, R.G., Hunt, K.J., Hazuda, H.P., and Stern, M.P. (2008). Fueling the obesity epidemic? Artificially sweetened beverage use and long-term weight gain. Obesity (Silver Spring) *16*, 1894-1900.

3. Sansom, W. (2005). New analysis suggests 'diet soda paradox' -- less sugar, more weight. In HSC News (San Antonio).

4. Swithers, S.E., and Davidson, T.L. (2008). A role for sweet taste: calorie predictive relations in energy regulation by rats. Behav Neurosci *122*, 161-173.

5. Davidson, T.L., and Swithers, S.E. (2004). A Pavlovian approach to the problem of obesity. International Journal of Obesity *28*, 933-935.

6. Dams, L. (1978). Bees and honey-hunting scenes in the Mesolithic rock art of eastern Spain. Bee World *59*, 45-53.

7. Halacy, D., Jr. (1967). Science and Serendipity: Great Discoveries by Accident (Philadelphia: Macrea Smith Company).

8. Descottes, B. (2009). Cicatrisation par le miel, l'experience de 25 annees. Phytotherapie *7*, 112-116.

9. Fitzmaurice, S.D., Sivamani, R.K., and Isseroff, R.R. (2011). Antioxidant therapies for wound healing: a clinical guide to currently commercially available products. Skin Pharmacology & Physiology *24*, 113-126.

10. Eddy, J.J., and Gideonsen, M.D. (2005). Topical honey for diabetic foot ulcers. J Fam Pract *54*, 533-535.

11. Eddy, J.J., Gideonsen, M.D., and Mack, G.P. (2008). Practical considerations of using topical honey for neuropathic diabetic foot ulcers: a review. WMJ *107*, 187-190.

12. Molan, P.C., and Betts, J.A. (2008). Using honey to heal diabetic foot ulcers. Adv Skin Wound Care *21*, 313-316.

13. Lee, D.S., Sinno, S., and Khachemoune, A. (2011). Honey and wound healing: an overview. Am J Clin Dermatol *12*, 181-190.

## Chapter 1

1. Ransome, H.M. (1937). The Sacred Bee in Ancient Times and Folklore (London: George Allen and Unwin). pp. 91-92

2   Economic Research Service. U.S. Consumption of Caloric Sweeteners (USDA).

3   Bente, L., and Gerrior, S.A. (2002). Selected Food and Nutrient Highlights of the 20th Century: U.S. Food Supply Series, U.S. Department of Agriculture, Center for Nutrition Policy and Promotion, ed.

4   Moeller, S.M., Fryhofer, S.A., Osbahr, A.J., 3rd, and Robinowitz, C.B. (2009). The effects of high fructose syrup. Journal of the American College of Nutrition *28*, 619-626.

5   White, J.S. (2008). Straight talk about high-fructose corn syrup: what it is and what it ain't. Am J Clin Nutr *88*, 1716S-1721S.

6   Brown, C.M., Dulloo, A.G., and Montani, J.P. (2008). Sugary drinks in the pathogenesis of obesity and cardiovascular diseases. International Journal of Obesity *32 Suppl 6*, S28-34.

7   Fournier, P., and Dupuis, Y. (1975). Modulation of intestinal absorption of calcium. Journal de Physiologie (Paris) *70*, 479-491.

8   National Osteoporosis Foundation (2011). National Osteoporosis Fast Facts.

9   Chepulis, L.M. (2007). The effects of honey compared with sucrose and sugar-free diet on neutrophil phagocytosis and lymphocyte numbers after long-term feeding in rats. Journal of Complementary and Integrative Medicine *4*, Article 8.

10  Gheldof, N., Wang, X.-H., and Engeseth, N.J. (2002). Identification and quantification of antioxidant components of honeys from various floral sources. J Agric Food Chem *50*, 5870-5877.

11  Frank, R. (2005). Honig: köstlich und gesund [Honey: delicious and healthy] (Stuttgart: Ulmer).

12  National Honey Board. Honey: A Reference Guide to Nature's Sweetener. (Longmont, CO: National Honey Board), ibid.

13  Miraglio, A. (2002). Honey--Health and Therapeutic Qualities (Longmont, CO: The National Honey Board). pp. 3

14  Ibid. pp. 16

15  Engeseth, N.J. (2008). Telephone interview, K. Traynor, ed.

16  Gheldof, N., Wang, X.-H., and Engeseth, N.J. (2002). Identification and quantification of antioxidant components of honeys from various floral sources. J Agric Food Chem *50*, 5870-5877.

17  Gheldof, N., and Engeseth, N.J. Ibid.Antioxidant capacity of honeys from various floral sources based on the determination of oxygen radical absorbance capacity and inhibition of *in vitro* lipoprotein oxidation in human serum samples. 3050-3055.

18  Gheldof, N., Wang, X.-H., and Engeseth, N.J. Ibid.Identification and quantification of antioxidant components of honeys from various floral sources. 5870-5877.

19  Engeseth, N.J. (2008). Telephone interview, K. Traynor, ed.

20   Ibid.

21   McKibben, J., and Engeseth, N.J. (2002). Honey as a protective agent against lipid oxidation in ground turkey. J Agric Food Chem *50*, 592-595, Wang, X.H., Andrae, L., and Engeseth, N.J. Ibid.Antimutagenic effect of various honeys and sugars against Trp-p-1. 6923-6928.

22   Wang, X.H., Andrae, L., and Engeseth, N.J. (2002). Antimutagenic effect of various honeys and sugars against Trp-p-1. J Agric Food Chem *50*, 6923-6928.

23   Gheldof, N., and Engeseth, N.J. Ibid.Antioxidant capacity of honeys from various floral sources based on the determination of oxygen radical absorbance capacity and inhibition of *in vitro* lipoprotein oxidation in human serum samples. 3050-3055.

24   Ibid.

25   Gheldof, N., Wang, X.-H., and Engeseth, N.J. (2003). Buckwheat honey increases serum antioxidant capacity in humans. Ibid. *51*, 1500-1505.

26   Ibid.

27   Gheldof, N., and Engeseth, N.J. (2002). Antioxidant capacity of honeys from various floral sources based on the determination of oxygen radical absorbance capacity and inhibition of *in vitro* lipoprotein oxidation in human serum samples. Ibid. *50*, 3050-3055.

28   Bogdanov, S. (1989). Determination of pinocembrin in honey using HPLC. J Apic Res *28*, 55-57.

29   Gheldof, N., Wang, X.-H., and Engeseth, N.J. (2002). Identification and quantification of antioxidant components of honeys from various floral sources. J Agric Food Chem *50*, 5870-5877.

### INTERLUDE 1

1   Flower, B., and Rosenbaum, E. (1958). The Roman cookery book by Apicius (Londong: Geroge G. Harrap & Co.).

2   Grainger, S. (2007). The Myth of Apicius. Gastronomica: The Journal of Food and Culture *7*, 71-77.

3   Ibid. pp. 77

### CHAPTER 2

1   Huffman, T.N. (1983). The Trance Hypothesis and the Rock Art of Zimbabwe. South African Archaeological Society, Goodwin Series *4*, 49-53.

2   Cooke, C.K. (1971). Excavations in Zombepata Cave, Sipolilo District, Mashonaland, Rhodesia. South African Archaeological Bulletin *26*, 104-126.

3   Crane, E. (1999). The world history of beekeeping and honey hunting (London: Duckworth).

4   Ibid.

5   Forrest, R.D. (1982b). Early history of wound treatment. J R Soc Med *75*, 198-205.

6   Ibid.

7   Majno, G. (1975). The Healing Hand. Man and Wound in the Ancient World (Cambridge, Massachusetts: Harvard University Press).

8   Kramer, S.N., and Levey, M. (1955). The oldest medical text in man's recorded history: A Sumerian Physician's prescription book of 4000 years ago. In The Illustrated London News (London), pp. 370-371.

9   Webb, J.L. (1957). The oldest medical document. Bull Med Libr Assoc *45*, 1-4.

10  Ibid.

11  Kramer, S.N., and Levey, M. (1955). The oldest medical text in man's recorded history: A Sumerian Physician's prescription book of 4000 years ago. In The Illustrated London News (London), pp. 370-371. 371

12  Herold, E., and Leibold, G. (1991). Heilwerte aus dem Bienenvolk: Honig, Pollen, Gelee royale, Wachs, Propolis und Bienengift; ihre Bedeutung für die Gesundheit und Behandlung von Krankheiten. , Vol 12. Aufl (München: Ehrenwirth).

13  Majno, G. (1975). The Healing Hand. Man and Wound in the Ancient World (Cambridge, Massachusetts: Harvard University Press).

14  Parkinson, R. (1999). Cracking Codes: The Rosetta Stone and Decipherment (University of California Press).

15  Ibid.

16  Breasted, J. (1930). The Edwin Smith Surgical papyrus (facsimile and hieroglyphic transliteration with translation and commentary, in two volumes) (Chicago: The University of Chicago Press).

17  van Middendorp, J.J., Sanchez, G.M., and Burridge, A.L. (2010). The Edwin Smith papyrus: a clinical reappraisal of the oldest known document on spinal injuries. Eur Spine J *19*, 1815-1823.

18  Sanchez, G.M., and Burridge, A.L. (2007). Decision making in head injury management in the Edwin Smith Papyrus. Neurosurg Focus *23*, E5.

19  Majno, G. (1975). The Healing Hand. Man and Wound in the Ancient World (Cambridge, Massachusetts: Harvard University Press).

20  Pahor, A.L. (1992). Ear, nose and throat in Ancient Egypt. J Laryngol Otol *106*, 773-779.

21  Majno, G. (1975). The Healing Hand. Man and Wound in the Ancient World (Cambridge, Massachusetts: Harvard University Press).

22  Nunn, J.F. (1996). Ancient Egyptian medicine (University of Oklahoma Press).

23  Crane, E. (1999). The world history of beekeeping and honey hunting (London: Duckworth).

24  Ransome, H.M. (1937). The Sacred Bee in Ancient Times and Folklore (London: George Allen and Unwin). pp. 28

25 Majno, G. (1975). The Healing Hand. Man and Wound in the Ancient World (Cambridge, Massachusetts: Harvard University Press). 484

26 Pahor, A.L. (1992). Ear, nose and throat in Ancient Egypt. J Laryngol Otol *106*, 773-779.

27 Ruiz, A. (2001). The Spirit of Ancient Eygpt (New York: Algora).

28 Smith, L. (2011). The Kahun Gynaecological Papyrus: ancient Egyptian medicine. J Fam Plann Reprod Health Care *37*, 54-55.

29 Ibid.

30 Nunn, J.F. (1996). Ancient Egyptian medicine (University of Oklahoma Press).

31 Smith, L. (2011). The Kahun Gynaecological Papyrus: ancient Egyptian medicine. J Fam Plann Reprod Health Care *37*, 54-55.

32 Martinetto, P., Dooryhee, E., Anne, M., Talabot, J., Tsoucaris, G., and Walter, P.H. (1999). Cosmetic recipes and make-up manufacturing in ancient Egypt. ESRF *April*.

33 Majno, G. (1975). The Healing Hand. Man and Wound in the Ancient World (Cambridge, Massachusetts: Harvard University Press). 112

34 Nunn, J.F. (1996). Ancient Egyptian medicine (University of Oklahoma Press).

35 Jones, R. (2001). Honey and healing through ages. Honey and Healing. P. Munn and R. Jones. Cardiff, International Bee Research Association: 1-4. Pg. 1

36 Raju, V.K. (2003). Susruta of ancient India. . Indian Journal of Ophthalmology *51*, 119-122.

37 Loukas, M., Lanteri, A., Ferrauiola, J., Tubbs, R.S., Maharaja, G., Shoja, M.M., Yadav, A., and Rao, V.C. (2010). Anatomy in ancient India: a focus on the Susruta Samhita. J Anat *217*, 646-650.

38 Bhishagratna, K. (1907). An English Translation of the Sushruta Samhita based on original Sanskrit text (Calcutta).

39 Saraf, S., and Parihar, R.S. (2007). Sushruta: The first Plastic Surgeon in 600 B.C. The Internet Journal of Plastic Surgery *4*.

40 Loukas, M., Lanteri, A., Ferrauiola, J., Tubbs, R.S., Maharaja, G., Shoja, M.M., Yadav, A., and Rao, V.C. (2010). Anatomy in ancient India: a focus on the Susruta Samhita. J Anat *217*, 646-650.

41 Twain, M. (1898). Following the Equator: A Journey around the World (Hartford: The American Publishing Company). Pg. 480

42 Saraf, S., and Parihar, R.S. (2007). Sushruta: The first Plastic Surgeon in 600 B.C. The Internet Journal of Plastic Surgery *4*.

43 Bhishagratna, K. (1907). An English Translation of the Sushruta Samhita based on original Sanskrit text (Calcutta), ibid.

44 Raju, V.K. (2003). Susruta of ancient India. . Indian Journal of Ophthalmology *51*, 119-122.

45 Ibid.

46 Udwadia, T.E. (2011). Ghee and Honey Dressing for Infected Wounds. Indian

J Surg *73*, 278–283.

47 Bhishagratna, K. (1907). An English Translation of the Sushruta Samhita based on original Sanskrit text (Calcutta).

48 Ibid.

49 Ibid.

50 Ibid.

51 Loukas, M., Lanteri, A., Ferrauiola, J., Tubbs, R.S., Maharaja, G., Shoja, M.M., Yadav, A., and Rao, V.C. (2010). Anatomy in ancient India: a focus on the Susruta Samhita. J Anat *217*, 646-650.

52 Whitaker, I.S., Karoo, R.O., Spyrou, G., and Fenton, O.M. (2007). The birth of plastic surgery: the story of nasal reconstruction from the Edwin Smith Papyrus to the twenty-first century. Plast Reconstr Surg *120*, 327-336.

53 Ibid.

54 Ortiz-Monasterio, F., and Olmedo, A. (1981). Reconstruction of major nasal defects. Clin Plast Surg *8*, 565-586.

55 Majno, G. (1975). The Healing Hand. Man and Wound in the Ancient World (Cambridge, Massachusetts: Harvard University Press). 287

56 Hummer, K.E. (2010). *Rubus* Pharmacology: Antiquitity to the Present. Horticultural Science *45*, 1587-1591.

57 Rohde, E.S. (1922). The old English herbals (London: Longmans, Green and Co.).

58 Ibid. pp. 6.

59 Ibid. pp. 23

60 Crane, E. (1999). The world history of beekeeping and honey hunting (London: Duckworth). pp. 509

61 Rohde, E.S. (1922). The old English herbals (London: Longmans, Green and Co.). pp. 7.

62 Forrest, R.D. (1982a). Development of wound therapy from the Dark Ages to the present. J R Soc Med *75*, 268-273.

63 Forrest, R.D. (1982b). Early history of wound treatment. J R Soc Med *75*, 198-205.


## INTERLUDE 2

1 Oldershaw, R.L. (1998). Democritus - scientific wizard of the 5th century BC. Speculations in Science and Technology *21*, 37-44.

2 Lowell, J.R. (1867). A Great Public Character. In The Atlantic Monthly (Boston: Ticknor and Fields), pp. 625

3 Ransome, H.M. (1937). The Sacred Bee in Ancient Times and Folklore (London: George Allen and Unwin).

## CHAPTER 3

1   Crane, E. (1999). The world history of beekeeping and honey hunting (London: Duckworth). pp. 509

2   Majno, G. (1975). The Healing Hand. Man and Wound in the Ancient World (Cambridge, Massachusetts: Harvard University Press).

3   Sackett, W.G. (1919). Honey as a carrier of intestinal diseases. In Bull Colorado State Univ Agric Exp Stn, pp. 1-18.

4   Dustmann, J.H. (1979). Antibacterial effect of honey. Apiacta *14*, 7-11.

5   Dold, H., Du, D.H., and Dziao, S.T. (1937). Nachweis antibakterieller, hitze- und lichtempfindlicher Hemmungsstoffe Inhibine im Naturhonig Blütenhonig. Z Hyg Infektionskr *120*, 155-167.

6   Gould, I.M., and van der Meer, J.W.M. (2005). Antibiotic policies theory and practice (New York: Kluwer Academic/Plenum).

7   Shimanuki et al., ed. (2007) The ABC and XYZ of Bee Culture. 41$^{st}$ ed. A.I. Root Company. Medina OH.

8   Jonathan W. White, Jr. Papers, 1890-2000, MGN 335, Penn State University Archives, Special Collections Library, University Libraries, Pennsylvania State University.

9   Molan, P.C. (2001) Why honey is effective as a medicine 2. The scientific explanation of its effects. *Bee World* 82(1): 22-40

10  McKenna, M. (2010). Superbug: The Fatal Menace of MRSA (New York: Free Press).

11  Molan, P.C. (1992b). The antibacterial activity of honey. 2. Variation in the potency of the antibacterial activity. Bee World *73*, 59-76, White, J.W. (1975). Composition of honey. In Honey: a Comprehensive Survey, E. Crane, ed. (London: Heinemann), pp. 157-206.

12  Molan, P.C. (1992b). The antibacterial activity of honey. 2. Variation in the potency of the antibacterial activity. Bee World *73*, 59-76.

13  Dustmann, J.H. (1967). Messung von Wasserstoffperoxid und Enzymeaktivitaet in mitteleuropaeischen Honigen. Zeitschrift fuer Bienenforschung *9*, 66-73.

14  Molan, P.C. (1992b). The antibacterial activity of honey. 2. Variation in the potency of the antibacterial activity. Bee World *73*, 59-76.

15  Molan, P. (2008). An explanation of why the MGO level in manuka honey does not show the antibacterial activity. N Z Beekeeper *16*, 11-13. pp.12

16  Molan, P.C. (1992a). The antibacterial activity of honey. 1. The nature of the antibacterial activity. Bee World *73*, 5-28.

17  Brady, N.F., Molan, P.C., and Harfoot, C.G. (1997). The sensitivity of dermatophytes to the antimicrobial activity of manuka honey and other honey. Pharm Sci *2*, 1-3.

## Chapter 4

1   Danforth, B.N., Sipes, S., Fang, J., and Brady, S.G. (2006). The history of early bee diversification based on five genes plus morphology. Proc Nat Acad Sci USA 103, 15118-15123.

2   Donoghue, M.J. (2002). Plants. In Encyclopedia of Evolution, M. Pagel, ed. (Oxford University Press).

3   Snodgrass, R.E. (1935). Principles of Insect Morphology (New York: McGraw-Hill Co.).

4   Snodgrass, R.E. (1956). Anatomy of the Honey Bee (New York: Cornell University Press).

5   Winston, M.L. (1987). The biology of the honey bee (First Harvard University Press).

6   Bailey, L. (1952). The action of the proventriculus of the worker honeybee, Apis mellifera L. The Journal of Experimental Biology 29, 310-329.

7   Whitcomb, and Wilson, H.F. (1929). Mechanics of digestion of pollen by the adult honey bee and the relation of undigested parts to dysentry of bees. Agric exp Stn, Univ Wisconsin, Res Bull 92, 1-29.

8   Lindauer, M. (1954). *Temperaturregulierung Und Wasserhaushalt Im Bienenstaat. Z Vgl Physiol 36, 391-432.

9   Seeley, T.D. (1989). Social Foraging in Honey Bees - How Nectar Foragers Assess Their Colony Nutritional-Status. Behavioral Ecology and Sociobiology 24, 181-199.

10  Von der Ohe, W., Dustmann, J., and Von der Ohe, K. (1991). Proline als Kriterium der Reife des Honigs. Dtsch Lebensm-Rundsch 87, 383-386.

11  Olofsson, T.C., and Vasquez, A. (2008). Detection and Identification of a Novel Lactic Acid Bacterial Flora Within the Honey Stomach of the Honeybee Apis mellifera. Current Microbiology 57, 356-363.

12  Forsgren, E., Olofsson, T.C., Vasquez, A., and Fries, I. (2009). Novel lactic acid bacteria inhibiting Paenibacillus larvae in honey bee larvae. Apidologie 41, 99-108.

13  Snodgrass, R.E. (1956). Anatomy of the Honey Bee (New York: Cornell University Press).

## Part II

## Chapter 5

1   American Cancer Society (2008). Cancer Facts & Figures 2008 (Atlanta: American Cancer Society).

2   American Cancer Society (2011). Cancer Facts & Figures 2011 (Atlanta: American Cancer Society).

3   Ravandi-Kashani, F., and Hayes, T.G. (1998). Male breast cancer: a review of the literature. Eur J Cancer 34, 1341-1347.

4   Sanchez, G.M., and Burridge, A.L. (2007). Decision making in head injury management in the Edwin Smith Papyrus. Neurosurg Focus 23, E5.

5   National Cancer Institute. Fact Sheet: Psychological Stress and Cancer (National Cancer Institute).

6   American Cancer Society (2008). Cancer Facts & Figures 2008 (Atlanta: American Cancer Society), American Cancer Society (2011). Cancer Facts & Figures 2011 (Atlanta: American Cancer Society). p.1.

7   Biswal, B.M. (2008). RE: Topical application of honey in the management of radiation mucositis. A Preliminary study K.S. Traynor, ed.

8   Biswal, B.M., Zakaria, A., and Ahmad, N.M. (2003). Topical application of honey in the management of radiation mucositis: a preliminary study. Support Care Cancer 11, 242-248.

9   Motallebnejad, M., Akram, S., Moghadamnia, A., Moulana, Z., and Omidi, S. (2008). The effect of topical application of pure honey on radiation-induced mucositis: a randomized clinical trial. J Contemp Dent Pract 9, 40-47.

10  Biswal, B.M., Zakaria, A., and Ahmad, N.M. (2003). Topical application of honey in the management of radiation mucositis: a preliminary study. Support Care Cancer 11, 242-248.

11  Biswal, B.M. (2008). RE: Topical application of honey in the management of radiation mucositis. A Preliminary study K.S. Traynor, ed.

12  Ibid.

13  Ibid.

14  Ibid.

15  Jones, R. (2001). Honey and healing through ages. In Honey and Healing, P. Munn, and R. Jones, eds. (Cardiff: International Bee Research Association), pp. 1-4.

16  Motallebnejad, M., Akram, S., Moghadamnia, A., Moulana, Z., and Omidi, S. (2008). The effect of topical application of pure honey on radiation-induced mucositis: a randomized clinical trial. J Contemp Dent Pract 9, 40-47.

17  Ibid.

18  Sela, M., Maroz, D., and Gedalia, I. (2000). Streptococcus mutans in saliva of normal subjects and neck and head irradiated cancer subjects after consumption of honey. J Oral Rehab 27, 269-270.

19  Sela, M.O., Shapira, L., Grizim, I., Lewinstein, I., Steinberg, D., Gedalia, I., and Grobler, S.R. (1998). Effects of honey consumption on enamel microhardness in normal versus xerostomic patients. J Oral Rehabil 25, 630-634.

20  Zidan, J., Shetver, L., Gershuny, A., Abzah, A., Tamam, S., Stein, M., and Friedman, E. (2006). Prevention of chemotherapy-induced neutropenia by special honey intake. Med Oncol 23, 549-552.

21  Simon, A., Sofka, K., Wiszniewsky, G., Blaser, G., Bode, U., and Fleischhack, G. (2006). Wound care with antibacterial honey (Medihoney) in pediatric

hematology-oncology. Support Care Cancer 14, 91-97.

22  Simon, Arne. Personal Interview at the Kinderklinik in Bonn, Germany on Feb. 15th, 2007.

23  Simon, A., Sofka, K., Wiszniewsky, G., Blaser, G., Bode, U., and Fleischhack, G. (2006). Wound care with antibacterial honey (Medihoney) in pediatric hematology-oncology. Support Care Cancer 14, 91-97.

24  Moolenaar, M., Poorter, R.L., van der Toorn, P.P., Lenderink, A.W., Poortmans, P., and Egberts, A.C. (2006). The effect of honey compared to conventional treatment on healing of radiotherapy-induced skin toxicity in breast cancer patients. Acta Oncol 45, 623-624.

25  Ibid.

26  Stein, J. (2011). Manuka Honey Shows Potential For Radiation-Induced Dermatitis (Medical News Today).

27  Ramirez, P.T., Wolf, J.K., and Levenback, C. (2003). Laparoscopic port-site metastases: etiology and prevention. Gynecol Oncol 91, 179-189.

28  Hamzaoglu, I., Saribeyoglu, K., Durak, H., Karahasanoglu, T., Bayrak, I., Altug, T., Sirin, F., and Sariyar, M. (2000). Protective covering of surgical wounds with honey impedes tumor implantation. Arch Surg 135, 1414-1417.

29  Ibid.

30  Mustoe, T.A. Ibid.Protective covering of surgical wounds with honey impedes tumor implantation--invited critique. 1417.

31  Johnson, D.W., van Eps, C., Mudge, D.W., Wiggins, K.J., Armstrong, K., Hawley, C.M., Campbell, S.B., Isbel, N.M., Nimmo, G.R., and Gibbs, H. (2005). Randomized, controlled trial of topical exit-site application of honey (Medihoney) versus mupirocin for the prevention of catheter-associated infections in hemodialysis patients. J Am Soc Nephrol 16, 1456-1462.

32  National Cancer Institute (2010). What you need to know about bladder cancer (National Institute of Health,).

33  Swellam, T., Miyanaga, N., Onozawa, M., Hattori, K., Kawai, K., Shimazui, T., and Akaza, H. (2003). Antineoplastic activity of honey in an experimental bladder cancer implantation model: in vivo and in vitro studies. Int J Urol 10, 213-219.

34  Ibid.

## CHAPTER 6

1  Centers for Disease Control and Prevention (2011). National diabetes fact sheet: national estimates and general information on diabetes and prediabetes in the United States, 2011, U.S. Department of Health and Human Services, ed. (Atlanta, GA: Centers for Disease Control and Prevention).

2  Ibid., National Institute of Diabetes and Digestive and Kidney Diseases (2005). National Diabetes Statistics fact sheet: general information and national estimates on diabetes in the United States, 2005, U.S. Department of

Health and Human Services, National Institute of Health, ed. (Bethesda, MD: National Institute of Health).

3    Baer, D. (2008). The Challenges of Insulin Resistance and Diabetes—Does Honey Play a Role. In International Symposium on Honey and Human Health (Sacramento, CA).

4    National Institute of Diabetes and Digestive and Kidney Diseases (2005). National Diabetes Statistics fact sheet: general information and national estimates on diabetes in the United States, 2005, U.S. Department of Health and Human Services, National Institute of Health, ed. (Bethesda, MD: National Institute of Health).

5    Centers for Disease Control and Prevention (2011). National diabetes fact sheet: national estimates and general information on diabetes and prediabetes in the United States, 2011, U.S. Department of Health and Human Services, ed. (Atlanta, GA: Centers for Disease Control and Prevention).

6    National Institute of Diabetes and Digestive and Kidney Diseases (2005). National Diabetes Statistics fact sheet: general information and national estimates on diabetes in the United States, 2005, U.S. Department of Health and Human Services, National Institute of Health, ed. (Bethesda, MD: National Institute of Health).

7    Center for Disease Control and Prevention (2004). National diabetes fact sheet: general information and national estimates on diabetes in the United States, 2003, U.S. Department of Health and Human Services, ed. (Atlanta, GA: Centers for Disease Control and Prevention).

8    Baer, D. (2008). The Challenges of Insulin Resistance and Diabetes—Does Honey Play a Role. In International Symposium on Honey and Human Health (Sacramento, CA).

9    Centers for Disease Control and Prevention (2011). National diabetes fact sheet: national estimates and general information on diabetes and prediabetes in the United States, 2011, U.S. Department of Health and Human Services, ed. (Atlanta, GA: Centers for Disease Control and Prevention).

10   National Institute of Diabetes and Digestive and Kidney Diseases (2005). National Diabetes Statistics fact sheet: general information and national estimates on diabetes in the United States, 2005, U.S. Department of Health and Human Services, National Institute of Health, ed. (Bethesda, MD: National Institute of Health).

11   Sinha, R., Fisch, G., Teague, B., Tamborlane, W.V., Banyas, B., Allen, K., Savoye, M., Rieger, V., Taksali, S., Barbetta, G., et al. (2002). Prevalence of impaired glucose tolerance among children and adolescents with marked obesity. N Engl J Med 346, 802-810.

12   Al-Waili, N.S. (2004). Natural honey lowers plasma glucose, C-reactive protein, homocysteine, and blood lipids in healthy, diabetic, and hyperlipidemic subjects: Comparison with dextrose and sucrose. J Med Food 7, 100-107.

13  Shambaugh, P., Worthington, V., and Herbert, J.H. (1990). Differential effects of honey, sucrose, and fructose on blood sugar levels. J Manipulative Physiol Ther 13, 322-325.

14  Samanta, A., Burden, A.C., and Jones, G.R. (1985). Plasma glucose responses to glucose, sucrose, and honey in patients with diabetes mellitus: an analysis of glycaemic and peak incremental indices. Diabetic Med 2, 371-373.

15  Shambaugh, P., Worthington, V., and Herbert, J.H. (1990). Differential effects of honey, sucrose, and fructose on blood sugar levels. J Manipulative Physiol Ther 13, 322-325.

16  Samanta, A., Burden, A.C., and Jones, G.R. (1985). Plasma glucose responses to glucose, sucrose, and honey in patients with diabetes mellitus: an analysis of glycaemic and peak incremental indices. Diabetic Med 2, 371-373.

17  Baer, D. (2008). The Challenges of Insulin Resistance and Diabetes—Does Honey Play a Role. In International Symposium on Honey and Human Health (Sacramento, CA).

18  Ionescu-Tirgoviste, C., Popa, E., Sintu, E., Mihalache, N., Cheta, D., and Mincu, I. (1983). Blood glucose and plasma insulin responses to various carbohydrates in type 2 (non-insulin-dependent) diabetes. Diabetologia 24, 80-84.

19  Gheldof, N., Wang, X.-H., and Engeseth, N.J. (2003). Buckwheat honey increases serum antioxidant capacity in humans. J Agric Food Chem 51, 1500-1505.

20  Berenbaum, M. (2008). Interview with May Berenbaum on antioxidants in honey, K. Traynor, ed.

21  Frankel, S., Robinson, G.E., and Berenbaum, M.R. (1998). Antioxidant capacity and correlated characteristics of 14 unifloral honeys. J Apic Res 37, 27-31.

22  Berenbaum, M. (2008). Interview with May Berenbaum on antioxidants in honey, K. Traynor, ed.

23  Ionescu-Tirgoviste, C., Popa, E., Sintu, E., Mihalache, N., Cheta, D., and Mincu, I. (1983). Blood glucose and plasma insulin responses to various carbohydrates in type 2 (non-insulin-dependent) diabetes. Diabetologia 24, 80-84.

24  Chepulis, L., and Starkey, N. (2008). The long-term effects of feeding honey compared with sucrose and a sugar-free diet on weight gain, lipid profiles, and DEXA measurements in rats. J Food Sci 73, H1-7.

25  Sweitzer, S.M., Fann, S.A., Borg, T.K., Baynes, J.W., and Yost, M.J. (2006). What is the future of diabetic wound care? The Diabetes Educator 32, 197-210.

26  Molan, P.C., and Betts, J.A. (2008). Using honey to heal diabetic foot ulcers. Advances in Skin & Wound Care 21, 313-316.

27  Pierre, E.J., Barrow, R.E., Hawkins, H.K., Nguyen, T.T., Sakurai, Y., Desai, M., Wolfe, R.R., and Herndon, D.N. (1998). Effects of insulin on wound

healing. J Trauma Injury Infect Crit Care 44, 342-345.

28  Belfield, W.O., Golinsky, S., and Compton, M.D. (1970). The use of insulin in open wound healing. Vet Med Small Anim Clin 65, 455-460.

29  Lopez, J.E., and Mena, B. (1968). Local insulin for diabetic gangrene. Lancet i, 1199.

30  Al-Waili, N. (2003). Intrapulmonary administration of natural honey solution, hyperosmolar dextrose or hypoosmolar distill water to normal individuals and to patients with type-2 diabetes mellitus or hypertension: their effects on blood glucose level, plasma insulin and C-peptide, blood pressure and peaked expiratory flow rate. Eur J Med Res 8, 295-303.

31  Molan, P.C. (2006). The evidence supporting the use of honey as a wound dressing. The International Journal of Lower Extremity Wounds 5, 40-54.

## CHAPTER 7

1  Center for Disease Control and Prevention (2008). Fast Stats A to Z: Allergies/Hay Fever.

2  Croft, L.R. (1990). Honey and Hay Fever (Salford, England: University of Salford).

3  American Academy of Allergy, Asthma and Immunology (2008). Allergy Statistics.

4  Hill, J. (1989). The virtues of honey (Chorley, Lancashire: Elmwood Books).

5  Croft, L.R. (1990). Honey and Hay Fever (Salford, England: University of Salford).

6  Ibid.

## CHAPTER 8

1  Paul, I.M., Beiler, J., McMonagle, A., Shaffer, M.L., Duda, L., and Berlin, C.M.J. (2007). Effect of honey, dextromethorphan, and no treatment on nocturnal cough and sleep quality for coughing children and their parents. Arch Pediatr Adolesc Med 161, 1140-1146.

2  Pfeiffer, W.F. (2005). A multicultural approach to the patient who has a common cold. Pediatr Rev 26, 170-175.

3  World Health Organization (2001). Cough and cold remedies for the treatment of acute respiratory infections in young children., Department of child and adolescent health and development., ed. (Geneva, Switzerland: World Health Organization), pp. 43.

4  Beiler, J. (2008). Honey as a Cough Suppressant. In International Symposium on Honey and Human Health (Sacramento, CA).

5  Paul, I.M., Yoder, K.E., Crowell, K.R., Shaffer, M.L., McMillan, H.S., Carlson, L.C., Dilworth, D.A., and Berlin, C.M., Jr. (2004). Effect of dextromethorphan, diphenhydramine, and placebo on nocturnal cough and

sleep quality for coughing children and their parents. Pediatrics 114, e85-90.

6 Anon. (1997). Use of codeine- and dextromethorphan-containing cough remedies in children. American Academy of Pediatrics. Committee on Drugs. Ibid. 99, 918-920.

7 Chang, A.B., and Glomb, W.B. (2006). Guidelines for evaluating chronic cough in pediatrics: ACCP evidence-based clinical practice guidelines. Chest 129, 260S-283S.

8 Center for Disease Control and Prevention (2005). Infant Deaths Associated with Cough and Cold Medications, Center for Disease Control and Prevention, ed. (MMWR), pp. 1-4.

9 World Health Organization (2001). Cough and cold remedies for the treatment of acute respiratory infections in young children., Department of child and adolescent health and development., ed. (Geneva, Switzerland: World Health Organization), pp. 43.

10 Pfeiffer, W.F. (2005). A multicultural approach to the patient who has a common cold. Pediatr Rev 26, 170-175.

11 Paul, I.M., Beiler, J., McMonagle, A., Shaffer, M.L., Duda, L., and Berlin, C.M.J. (2007). Effect of honey, dextromethorphan, and no treatment on nocturnal cough and sleep quality for coughing children and their parents. Arch Pediatr Adolesc Med 161, 1140-1146.

12 U.S. Food and Drug Administration (2008). FDA Releases Recommendations Regarding Use of Over-the-Counter Cough and Cold Products; Products should not be used in children under 2 years of age; evaluation continues in older populations, U.S. Food and Drug Administration, ed.

## CHAPTER 9

1 Salminen, S., Gueimonde, M., and Isolauri, E. (2005). Probiotics that modify disease. J Nutrition 135, 1294-1298.

2 Ibid.

3 Guarner F, Schaafsma GJ. Probiotics. Int J. Food Microbiol 1998; 39:237-8. quoted in Adolfsson et al. Yogurt and Gut Function. American Jounral of Clinical Nutrition 2004; 80:245-56. pg 245.

4 Chick, H., Shin, H.S., and Ustunol, Z. (2001). Growth and acid production by lactic acid bacteria and bifidobacteria grown in skim milk containing honey. J Food Sci 66, 478-481.

5 Ibid.

6 Molan, Peter. Email communication discussing honey and diarrhea from 12 April, 2007.

7 Kajiwara, S., Gandhi, H., and Ustunol, Z. (2002). Effect of honey on the growth of and acid production by human intestinal Bifidobacterium spp.: an in vitro comparison with commercial oligosaccharides and inulin. J Food Prot 65, 214-218.

8    Chick, H., Shin, H.S., and Ustunol, Z. (2001). Growth and acid production by lactic acid bacteria and bifidobacteria grown in skim milk containing honey. J Food Sci 66, 478-481.

9    Olofsson, T.C., and Vasquez, A. (2008). Detection and Identification of a Novel Lactic Acid Bacterial Flora Within the Honey Stomach of the Honeybee Apis mellifera. Current Microbiology 57, 356-363.

10   Ibid.

11   Rooney, P. (2008). One of the World's Sweetest Pleasures. In Western Mail.

12   Ustunol, Z., and Gandhi, H. (2001). Growth and viability of commercial Bifidobacterium spp. in honey-sweetened skim milk. J Food Prot 64, 1775-1779.

## CHAPTER 10

1    Starkey, N. (2008b). The Effect of Honey Compared to Sucrose, Mixed Sugars, and a Sugar-free Diet on Weight Gain in Young Rats. In International Symposium on Honey and Human Health (Sacramento, CA).

2    Chepulis, L., and Starkey, N. (2008). The long-term effects of feeding honey compared with sucrose and a sugar-free diet on weight gain, lipid profiles, and DEXA measurements in rats. J Food Sci 73, H1-7.

3    Starkey, N. (2008a). Cognitive Function: Mental Performance and Memory – Does Honey have a Role in Improving Human Cognition? In International Symposium on Honey and Human Health (Sacramento, CA).

4    Bogdanov, S., Jurendic, T., Sieber, R., and Gallmann, P. (2008). Honey for nutrition and health: a review. Journal of the American College of Nutrition 27, 677-689.

5    Chepulis, L., and Starkey, N. (2008). The long-term effects of feeding honey compared with sucrose and a sugar-free diet on weight gain, lipid profiles, and DEXA measurements in rats. J Food Sci 73, H1-7.

6    American Heart Association (2011). Good vs. Bad Cholesterol.

7    Frank, G.K., Oberndorfer, T.A., Simmons, A.N., Paulus, M.P., Fudge, J.L., Yang, T.T., and Kaye, W.H. (2008). Sucrose activates human taste pathways differently from artificial sweetener. Neuroimage 39, 1559-1569.

8    Davidson, T. and Swithers, S. (2008) "A Pavlovian Approach to Obesity"

9    Swithers, S.E., and Davidson, T.L. (2008). A role for sweet taste: calorie predictive relations in energy regulation by rats. Behav Neurosci 122, 161-173.

## CHAPTER 11

1    Chepulis, L.M. (2007). The effects of honey compared with sucrose and sugar-free diet on neutrophil phagocytosis and lymphocyte numbers after long-term feeding in rats. Journal of Complementary and Integrative Medicine 4, Article 8.

2 Zidan, J., Shetver, L., Gershuny, A., Abzah, A., Tamam, S., Stein, M., and Friedman, E. (2006). Prevention of chemotherapy-induced neutropenia by special honey intake. Med Oncol 23, 549-552.

3 Abuharfeil, N., Al-Oran, R., and Abo-Shehada, M. (1999). The effect of bee honey on proliferative activity of human B- and T-lymphocytes and the activity of phagocytes. Food Agric Immunol 11, 169-177.

4 Al-Waili, N.S., and Haq, A. (2004). Effect of honey on antibody production against thymus-dependent and thymus-independent antigens in primary and secondary immune responses. J Med Food 7, 491-494.

5 Chepulis, L.M. (2007). The effects of honey compared with sucrose and sugar-free diet on neutrophil phagocytosis and lymphocyte numbers after long-term feeding in rats. Journal of Complementary and Integrative Medicine 4, Article 8.

6 Ibid.

7 Starkey, N. (2008). Cognitive Function: Mental Performance and Memory – Does Honey have a Role in Improving Human Cognition? In International Symposium on Honey and Human Health (Sacramento, CA).

8 Al-Waili, N.S. (2003). Effects of daily consumption of honey solution on hematological indices and blood levels of minerals and enzymes in normal individuals. J Med Food 6, 135-140.

9 Gheldof, N., Wang, X.-H., and Engeseth, N.J. (2003). Buckwheat honey increases serum antioxidant capacity in humans. J Agric Food Chem 51, 1500-1505.

10 Schramm, D.D., Karim, M., Schrader, H.R., Holt, R.R., Cardetti, M., and Keen, C.L. Ibid.Honey with high levels of antioxidants can provide protection to healthy human subjects. 1732-1735.

## INTERLUDE 4

1 Jones, R. (2001). Honey and healing through ages. In Honey and Healing, P. Munn, and R. Jones, eds. (Cardiff: International Bee Research Association), pp. 1-4.

## CHAPTER 12

1 Aristotle, Historia animalium. 9, 27 quoted in Deissenberg, H. (1988). Botinnen der Götter: Natur- und Kulturgeschichte der Honigbiene (Rheinland Verlag).

2 Fotidar, M.R., and Fotidar, S.N. (1945). 'Lotus' honey. Indian Bee J 7, 102.

3 Sarma, M.C. (1988). Honey in the treatment of bacterial corneal ulcers. Personal communication cited in Efem, S. E. E.; Udoh, K. T.; Iwara, C. I. (1992) The antimicrobial spectrum of honey and its clinical significance. Infection 20(4):227-229.

4    Imperato, P.J., and Traoré, D. (1969). Traditional beliefs about measles and its treatment among the Bambara of Mali. Trop Geogr Med 21, 62-67.

5    Kello, A.B., and Gilbert, C. (2003). Causes of severe visual impairment and blindness in children in schools for the blind in Ethiopia. British Journal of Ophthalmology 87, 526-530.

6    Traynor, J. (2002). Honey: The Gourmet Medicine (Bakersfield, CA: Kovak Books). pp. 24

7    A Subscriber (1937). Am Bee J 77, p. 350.

8    Vit, P., Medina, M., and Enriquez, M.E. (2004). Quality standards for medicinal uses of Meliponinae honey in Guatemala, Mexico and Venezuela. Bee World 85, 2-5.

9    World Health Organisation (2011). Visual impairment and blindness, Fact Sheet No 282, W.H. Organisation, ed.

10   Ibid.

11   Vit, P., and Jacob, T.J. (2008). Putative Anticataract Properties of Honey Studied by the Action of Flavonoids on a Lens Culture Model. Journal of Health Science 54, 196-202.

12   Kupfer, C. (1985). Bowman lecture. The conquest of cataract: a global challenge. Trans Ophthalmol Soc U K 104 ( Pt 1), 1-10.

13   Vit, P. (2001). Stingless bee honey and the treatment of cataracts. In Honey and healing, P. Munn, and J. R., eds. (Cardiff: International Bee Research Association), pp. 37-40.

14   Vit, P., and Jacob, T.J. (2008). Putative Anticataract Properties of Honey Studied by the Action of Flavonoids on a Lens Culture Model. Journal of Health Science 54, 196-202.

15   Vit, P. (2001). Stingless bee honey and the treatment of cataracts. In Honey and healing, P. Munn, and J. R., eds. (Cardiff: International Bee Research Association), pp. 37-40.

16   Vit, P., and Jacob, T.J. (2008). Putative Anticataract Properties of Honey Studied by the Action of Flavonoids on a Lens Culture Model. Journal of Health Science 54, 196-202.

17   Yoirish, N. (1977). Curative Properties of Honey & Bee Venom (San Francisco: New Glide Publications).

18   Golychev, V.N. (1990). [Use of honey in conservative treatment of senile cataracts]. Vestn Oftalmol 106, 59-62.

19   Emarah, M.H. (1982). A clinical study of the topical use of bee honey in the treatment of some ocular diseases. Bull Islamic Med 2, 422-425.

20   Albietz, J.M., and Lenton, L.M. (2006). Effect of antibacterial honey on the ocular flora in tear deficiency and meibomian gland disease. Cornea 25, 1012-1019.

## Chapter 13

1   Strauss, M.B. (1968). Familiar Medical Quotations (Boston: Little Brown). pp. 65.

2   Fikree, F.F., Ali, T.S., Durocher, J.M., and Rahbar, M.H. (2005). Newborn care practices in low socioeconomic settlements of Karachi, Pakistan. Soc Sci Med 60, 911-921.

3   Celsus ((c.25 A.D.) 1935). De Medicina, Vol 2 (London: Heinemann). Prooemium 26

4   Ibid.Book II 29.

## Chapter 14

1   Celsus ((c.25 A.D.) 1935). De Medicina, Vol 2 (London: Heinemann).Book II 30

2   Al-Bukhari, M. ((c. 740 A.D.) 1976). Sahih Al-Bukhari, Vol VII, Third, revised edn (Chicago: Kazi Publications).

3   Lim, M.L., and Wallace, M.R. (2004). Infectious diarrhea in history. Infectious Disease Clinics of North America 18, 261-274.

4   Haffejee, I.E., and Moosa, A. (1985). Honey in the treatment of infantile gastroenteritis. Br Med J 290, 1866-1867.

5   Molan, P.C. (1999). Why honey is effective as a medicine. 1. Its use in modern medicine. Bee World 80, 80-92.

6   Honey: its antibacterial action in the treatment of gastroenteritis. Glimpse 1985 Nov-Dec; 7(6): 1,8.

7   Haffejee, I.E., and Moosa, A. (1985). Honey in the treatment of infantile gastroenteritis. Br Med J 290, 1866-1867.

8   World Health Organisation (2004). Water, Sanitation and Hygiene Links to Health, FACTS AND FIGURES, World Health Organisation, ed.

9   World Health Organisation (1976). Treatment and Prevention of Dehydration in Diarrhoeal Diseases, pp. 31.

10  Haffejee, I.E., and Moosa, A. (1985). Honey in the treatment of infantile gastroenteritis. Br Med J 290, 1866-1867.

11  Molan, P.C. (2001). Why honey is effective as a medicine. 2. The scientific explanation of its effects. Bee World 82, 22-40.

12  Anon. (1985). Honey: its antibacterial action in the treatment of gastroenteritis. Glimpse 7, 1, 8.

13  Molan, P.C. (1997). Honey as an antimicrobial agent. In Bee Products: Properties, Applications and Apitherapy, A. Mizrahi, and Y. Lensky, eds. (New York: Plenum Press), pp. 27-37.

14  Linnett, P. (1996). Honey for equine diarrhoea. In Control and Therapy, pp. 906.

15 Molan, P.C. (2001). Why honey is effective as a medicine. 2. The scientific explanation of its effects. Bee World 82, 22-40.

16 Adolfsson et al. Yogurt and Gut Function. American Jounral of Clinical Nutrition 2004; 80:245-56.

17 Adolfsson et al. Yogurt and Gut Function. American Jounral of Clinical Nutrition 2004; 80:245-56. pg 250.

18 Ezz El-Arab, A.M., Girgis, S.M., Hegazy, E.M., and Abd El-Khalek, A.B. (2006). Effect of dietary honey on intestinal microflora and toxicity of mycotoxins in mice. BMC Complement Altern Med 6, 6.

19 Shamala, T.R., Jyothi, Y.S., and Saibaba, P. (2000). Stimulatory effect of honey on multiplication of lactic acid bacteria under in vitro and in vivo conditions. Lett Appl Microbiol 30, 453-455.

20 Carson, C.F., and Riley, T.V. (2003). Non-antibiotic therapies for infectious diseases. Commun Dis Intell 27 Suppl, S144-147.

21 Johnson-Henry, K. (2007). Honey and gastrointestinal disorders, K. Traynor, ed.

## INTERLUDE 5

1 Deissenberg, H. (1988). Botinnen der Götter: Natur- und Kulturgeschichte der Honigbiene (Rheinland Verlag).

2 Guthrie, D. (1945). A History of Medicine, Second edn (London: Thomas Nelson). p. 58

3 Yonge, C.D. (1854). Deipnosophists or Banquet of the Learned of Atheneus, Vol 1 (London: Henry G. Bohn). p 76

## CHAPTER 15

1 Rheinisches Museumsamt, Heindrichs, H., and Hohorst, B. (1988). Botinnen Der Götter: Natur- Und Kulturgeschichte Der Honigbiene (Rheinland-Verlag).

2 National Honey Board (2004). Honey's Nutrition and Health Facts. National Honey Board Fact Sheet.

3 Crane, E. (1999). The world history of beekeeping and honey hunting (London: Duckworth).

4 White, J.W. (1975). Composition of honey. In Honey: a Comprehensive Survey, E. Crane, ed. (London: Heinemann), pp. 157-206.

5 McInnes, M., McInnes, S., and Stanfield, M. (2007). The Hibernation Diet (Souvenier Press). p. 134

6 Earnest, C.P., Lancaster, S.L., Rasmussen, C.J., Kerksick, C.M., Lucia, A., Greenwood, M.C., Almada, A.L., Cowan, P.A., and Kreider, R.B. (2004). Low vs. high glycemic index carbohydrate gel ingestion during simulated 64-km

cycling time trial performance. J Strength Cond Res 18, 466-472.

## Chapter 16

1   Royal Society of Chemistry (2007). Royal Society of Chemistry's hangover avoidance and alleviation advice (London: Royal Society of Chemistry).

2   Wiese, J.G., Shlipak, M.G., and Browner, W.S. (2000). The alcohol hangover. Ann Intern Med 132, 897-902.

3   Swift, R., and Davidson, D. (1998). Alcohol hangover: mechanisms and mediators. Alcohol Health Res World 22, 54-60.

4   Ibid.

5   Ibid.

6   Brown, S.S., Forrest, J.A., and Roscoe, P. (1972). A controlled trial of fructose in the treatment of acute alcoholic intoxication. Lancet 2, 898-899.

7   Diamond, M. (2008). Honey for your Hangover, K. Traynor, ed.

8   Ibid.

9   Swift, R., and Davidson, D. (1998). Alcohol hangover: mechanisms and mediators. Alcohol Health Res World 22, 54-60.

10  Ibid.

11  Diamond, M. (2008). Honey for your Hangover, K. Traynor, ed.

12  Royal Society of Chemistry (2007). Royal Society of Chemistry's hangover avoidance and alleviation advice (London: Royal Society of Chemistry).

13  Swift, R., and Davidson, D. (1998). Alcohol hangover: mechanisms and mediators. Alcohol Health Res World 22, 54-60.

14  Royal Society of Chemistry (2007). Royal Society of Chemistry's hangover avoidance and alleviation advice (London: Royal Society of Chemistry).

15  Swift, R., and Davidson, D. (1998). Alcohol hangover: mechanisms and mediators. Alcohol Health Res World 22, 54-60.

## Chapter 17

1   Van Eaton, C. (2001). Botulism and honey. In Honey and healing, P. Munn, and R. Jones, eds. (Cardiff: International Bee Research Association), pp. 48-49.

2   Lawrence, W.B. (1986). Infant botulism and its relationship to honey: a review. Am Bee J 126, 484-486.

3   Crane, E. (1979). Honey in relation to infant botulism. Bee World 60, 152-154.

4   Ransome, H.M. (1937). The Sacred Bee in Ancient Times and Folklore (London: George Allen and Unwin). pp. 136

5   Ibid. pp. 160

6   Rhman, M.A., and Tayseer, N. (2005). Not giving honey to infants: A recommendation that should be reevaluated Journal of the American

Apitherapy Society.

7   Krell, R. (1996). Value-added products from beekeeping (Rome: Food and
    Agricultural Organization of the United Nations).

8   Bogdanov, S., Jurendic, T., Sieber, R., and Gallmann, P. (2008). Honey for
    nutrition and health: a review. Journal of the American College of Nutrition
    27, 677-689.

9   Takuma, D. (1955). Honig bei der Aufzucht von Säuglingen. Monatsschrift
    Kinderheilkunde 103, 160-161.

10  Maglietta, V. (1968). Sull'Impiego del Miel in Pediatria. Clin Pediatr (Bologna)
    50, 589-601.

11  Anon. (1965). La miel en la alimentación del lactante. Rev Esp Pediatr 21,
    333-340.

12  Mommsen, H. (1957). [Vitality of nutrition, a new concept of quality.].
    Hippokrates 28, 193-198.

13  Takuma, D. (1955). Honig bei der Aufzucht von Säuglingen. Monatsschrift
    Kinderheilkunde 103, 160-161.

14  Ramenghi, L.A., Amerio, G., and Sabatino, G. (2001). Honey, a palatable
    substance for infants: from De Rerum Natura to evidence-based medicine.
    European Journal of Pediatrics 160, 677-678.

15  Van Eaton, C. (2001). Botulism and honey. In Honey and healing, P. Munn,
    and R. Jones, eds. (Cardiff: International Bee Research Association), pp. 48-49.

16  Molan, P.C., and Allen, K.L. (1996). The effect of gamma-irradiation on the
    antibacterial activity of honey. J Pharm Pharmacol 48, 1206-1209.

17  Seymour, F.I., and West, K.S. (1951). Honey - its role in medicine. Med Times
    79, 104-107.


INTERLUDE 6

1   Paton, W.R. (1918). The Greek Anthology (London: William Heinemann).
    pp. 283

2    Calverley, C.S. (1869). Theocritus (Cambridge: Deighton, Bell, and Co.). pp.
    109


PART III

1   The names of the mother and child have been changed to protect the privacy
    of the family and the case history constructed from information presented in
    published papers and conversation with the attending physician.

2   Simon, A., Sofka, K., Wiszniewsky, G., Blaser, G., Bode, U., and Fleischhack,
    G. (2006). Wound care with antibacterial honey (Medihoney) in pediatric
    hematology-oncology. Support Care Cancer 14, 91-97. ibid.

3   Werner, S., and Grose, R. (2003). Regulation of wound healing by growth factors and cytokines. Physiol Rev 83, 835-870.

4   The name of the boy has been changed to protect the privacy of the family and the case history constructed from information presented in published papers and conversation with the attending physician.

5   Rice, L.B. (2006). Antimicrobial resistance in gram-positive bacteria. Am J Med 119, S11-19; discussion S62-70.

## CHAPTER 18

1   Polak, F., Clift, M., Bower, L., and Sprange, K. (2008). Buyers' guide: Advanced wound dressing, National Health Service: Centre for Evidence-based Purchasing, ed. (London).

2   Yang, K.L. (1944). The use of honey in the treatment of chilblains, non-specific ulcers, and small wounds. Chin Med J *62*, 55-60.

3   Bergman, A., Yanai, J., Weiss, J., Bell, D., and David, M.P. (1983). Acceleration of wound healing by topical application of honey. An animal model. Am J Surg *145*, 374-376.

4   Dunford C *et al.*(2000)The use of honey in wound management. *Nursing Standard*. 15, 11, 63-68.

5   Cooper, R.A., Molan, P.C., and Harding, K.G. (2002). The sensitivity to honey of Gram-positive cocci of clinical significance isolated from wounds. J Appl Microbiol *93*, 857-863.

6   Cooper, R. (2001). How does honey heal wounds? In Honey and healing, P. Munn, and R. Jones, eds. (Cardiff: International Bee Research Association), pp. 27-34.

7   Postmes, T., and Vandeputte, J. (1999). Recombinant growth factors or honey? Burns *25*, 676-678.

8   Davis, C., and Arnold, K. (1974). Role of meningococcal endotoxin in meningococcal purpura. J Exp Med *140*, 159-171.

9   Silver, I.A. (1980). The physiology of wound healing. In Wound healing and wound infection: theory and surgical practice, T.K. Hunt, ed. (New York: Appleton-Century-Crofts), pp. 11-28.

10  Molan, P.C. (1998). A brief review of honey as a clinical dressing. Primary Intention *6*, 148-158.

11  Jenkins, R., Burton, N., and Cooper, R. (2011). Manuka honey inhibits cell division in methicillin-resistant Staphylococcus aureus. J Antimicrob Chemother.

12  Molan, P.C. (2001). Why honey is effective as a medicine. 2. The scientific explanation of its effects. Bee World *82*, 22-40.

13  Molan, P.C. (2002). Re-introducing honey in the management of wounds and ulcers - theory and practice. Ostomy/Wound Manage *48*, 28-40.

14  White, R. (2005). The benefits of honey in wound management. Nurs Stand *20*, 57-64; quiz 66.

15  Frankel, S., Robinson, G.E., and Berenbaum, M.R. (1998). Antioxidant capacity and correlated characteristics of 14 unifloral honeys. J Apic Res *37*, 27-31.

16  Dailey, L.A., and Imming, P. (1999). 12-Lipoxygenase: classification, possible therapeutic benefits from inhibition, and inhibitors. Curr Med Chem *6*, 389-398.

17  Dunford, C.E., and Hanano, R. (2004). Acceptability to patients of a honey dressing for non-healing venous leg ulcers. J Wound Care *13*, 193-197.

18  Molan, P.C. (2002). Re-introducing honey in the management of wounds and ulcers - theory and practice. Ostomy/Wound Manage *48*, 28-40.

19  Pieper, B. (2009). Honey-based dressings and wound care: an option for care in the United States. J Wound Ostomy Continence Nurs *36*, 60-66; quiz 67-68.

20  DiPietro, L.A. (1995). Wound healing: the role of the macrophage and other immune cells. Shock *4*, 233-240.

21  Oryan, A., and Zaker, S.R. (1998). Effects of topical application of honey on cutaneous wound healing in rabbits. J Vet Med Ser A *45*, 181-188.

22  Molan, P.C. (2002). Re-introducing honey in the management of wounds and ulcers - theory and practice. Ostomy/Wound Manage *48*, 28-40.

23  Jones, K.P., Blair, S., Tonks, A., Price, A., and Cooper, R. (2000). Honey and the stimulation of inflammatory cytokine release from a monocytic cell line. Paper presented at: First World Wound Healing Congress (Melbourne, Australia).

24  Abuharfeil, N., Al-Oran, R., and Abo-Shehada, M. (1999). The effect of bee honey on proliferative activity of human B- and T-lymphocytes and the activity of phagocytes. Food Agric Immunol *11*, 169-177.

25  Molan, P.C. (2006). Using honey in wound care. International Journal of Clinical Aromatherapy *3*, 21-24.

26  Güneş, Ü.Y., and Eşer, I. (2007). Effectiveness of a honey dressing for healing pressure ulcers. J Wound Ostomy Continence Nurs *34*, 184-190.

27  Pieper, B. (2009). Honey-based dressings and wound care: an option for care in the United States. J Wound Ostomy Continence Nurs *36*, 60-66; quiz 67-68.

28  Gethin, G., and Cowman, S. (2005). Case series of use of Manuka honey in leg ulceration. Int Wound J *2*, 10-15.

29  Blaser, G., Santos, K., Bode, U., Vetter, H., and Simon, A. (2007). Effect of medical honey on wounds colonised or infected with MRSA. J Wound Care *16*, 325-328.

30  Dunford, C.E., and Hanano, R. (2004). Acceptability to patients of a honey dressing for non-healing venous leg ulcers. Ibid. *13*, 193-197.

31  Blaser, G., Santos, K., Bode, U., Vetter, H., and Simon, A. (2007). Effect of medical honey on wounds colonised or infected with MRSA. Ibid. *16*, 325-328.

32  Cunha, B.A. (2001). Antibiotic side effects. Medical Clinics of North America *85*, 149-185.

33  Molan, P.C. (2001). Honey as a topical antibacterial agent for treatment of infected wounds. World Wide Wounds, http://www.worldwidewounds. com/2001/november/Molan/honey-as-topical-agent.html.


INTERLUDE 7

1  Frazer, J.G. (1913). Pausanias's Description of Greece, Vol II (London: Macmillan and Co). pp. 424

2  National Honey Board Notable, Quotable Honey.


CHAPTER 19

1  The patient's name has been changed to protect the individual's identity and the case history constructed from information presented in the published paper and an interview with Dr. Eddy.

2  Eddy, J.J., and Gideonsen, M.D. (2005). Topical honey for diabetic foot ulcers. J Fam Pract 54, 533-535.

3  Eddy, J.J. (2008). Interview with Dr. Jennifer Eddy, K. Traynor, ed.

4  Majno, G. (1975). The Healing Hand. Man and Wound in the Ancient World (Cambridge, Massachusetts: Harvard University Press). 118.

5  Centers for Disease Control and Prevention (2011). National diabetes fact sheet: national estimates and general information on diabetes and prediabetes in the United States, 2011, U.S. Department of Health and Human Services, ed. (Atlanta, GA: Centers for Disease Control and Prevention).

6  Kleinfield, N.R. ( 2006 New York Times. ). Diabetes and Its Awful Toll Quietly Emerge as a Crisis. In New York Times (NY).

7  Center for Disease Control and Prevention (2004). National diabetes fact sheet: general information and national estimates on diabetes in the United States, 2003, U.S. Department of Health and Human Services, ed. (Atlanta, GA: Centers for Disease Control and Prevention).

8  Polak, F., Clift, M., Bower, L., and Sprange, K. (2008). Buyers' guide: Advanced wound dressing, National Health Service: Centre for Evidence-based Purchasing, ed. (London).

9  Gethin, G., and Cowman, S. (2009). Manuka honey vs. hydrogel--a prospective, open label, multicentre, randomised controlled trial to compare desloughing efficacy and healing outcomes in venous ulcers. J Clin Nurs 18, 466-474.

10   Gethin, G., and Cowman, S. (2005). Case series of use of Manuka honey in leg ulceration. Int Wound J 2, 10-15.

11   Ibid.

12   The patient's name has been changed to protect the individual's identity and the case history constructed from information presented in the published paper.

13   Gethin, G., and Cowman, S. (2005). Case series of use of Manuka honey in leg ulceration. Int Wound J 2, 10-15.

14   Gethin, G., and Cowman, S. (2009). Manuka honey vs. hydrogel--a prospective, open label, multicentre, randomised controlled trial to compare desloughing efficacy and healing outcomes in venous ulcers. J Clin Nurs 18, 466-474.

15   Gethin, G.T., Cowman, S., and Conroy, R.M. (2008). The impact of Manuka honey dressings on the surface pH of chronic wounds. Int Wound J 5, 185-194.

16   Jull, A., Walker, N., Parag, V., Molan, P., and Rodgers, A. (2008). Randomized clinical trial of honey-impregnated dressings for venous leg ulcers. Br J Surg 95, 175-182.

17   Dunford, C.E., and Hanano, R. (2004). Acceptability to patients of a honey dressing for non-healing venous leg ulcers. J Wound Care 13, 193-197.

18   Douglas, V. (2001). Living with a chronic leg ulcer: an insight into patients' experiences and feelings. Ibid. 10, 355-360.

19   Ibid.

20   Traynor, K. (2011). Interview with registered nurse Cheryl Dunford.

21   Douglas, V. (2001). Living with a chronic leg ulcer: an insight into patients' experiences and feelings. J Wound Care 10, 355-360.

22   Dunford, C. (2005). The use of honey in wound management. In Honey: A modern wound management product, R. White, R. Cooper, and P. Molan, eds. (Aberdeen, UK: Wounds UK Publishing), pp. 116-129.

23   Dunford, C.E., and Hanano, R. (2004). Acceptability to patients of a honey dressing for non-healing venous leg ulcers. J Wound Care 13, 193-197.

24   Van der Weyden, E.A. (2003). The use of honey for the treatment of two patients with pressure ulcers. Br J Community Nurs 8, S14-S20.

25   The patient's name has been changed to protect the individual's identity and the case history constructed from information presented in the published paper.

26   The patient's name has been changed to protect the individual's identity and the case history constructed from information presented in the published paper.

27   Van der Weyden, E.A. (2005). Treatment of a venous leg ulcer with a honey alginate dressing. Br J Community Nurs 10, S21, S24, S26-27.

28   Güneş, Ü.Y., and Eşer, I. (2007). Effectiveness of a honey dressing for healing

pressure ulcers. J Wound Ostomy Continence Nurs 34, 184-190.

29  Ibid.

## Chapter 20

1   The patient's name has been changed to protect the individual's identity and the case history constructed from information presented in the published paper.

2   Ahmed, A.K., Hoekstra, M.J., Hage, J.J., and Karim, R.B. (2003). Honey-medicated dressing: transformation of an ancient remedy into modern therapy. Ann Plast Surg 50, 143-147; discussion 147-148.

3   The patient's name has been changed to protect the individual's identity and the case history constructed from information presented in the published paper.

4   Ahmed, A.K., Hoekstra, M.J., Hage, J.J., and Karim, R.B. (2003). Honey-medicated dressing: transformation of an ancient remedy into modern therapy. Ann Plast Surg 50, 143-147; discussion 147-148.

5   Stephen-Haynes, J. (2004). Evaluation of a honey-impregnated tulle dressing in primary care. Br J Community Nurs 9, S21-27.

6   The patient's name has been changed to protect the individual's identity and the case history constructed from information presented in the published paper.

7   The patient's name has been changed to protect the individual's identity and the case history constructed from information presented in the published paper.

8   Stephen-Haynes, J. (2004). Evaluation of a honey-impregnated tulle dressing in primary care. Br J Community Nurs 9, S21-27, ibid.

9   Blaser, G., Santos, K., Bode, U., Vetter, H., and Simon, A. (2007). Effect of medical honey on wounds colonised or infected with MRSA. J Wound Care 16, 325-328.

10  The patient's name has been changed to protect the individual's identity and the case history constructed from information presented in the published paper.

11  As defined in the European Medical Device Directive: Council Directive 93/42/EEC of 14 June 1993

12  Vardi, A., Barzilay, Z., Linder, N., Cohen, H.A., Paret, G., and Barzilai, A. (1998). Local application of honey for treatment of neonatal postoperative wound infection. Acta Paediatr 87, 429-432.

13  Al-Waili, N.S., and Saloom, K.Y. (1999). Effects of topical honey on post-operative wound infections due to gram positive and gram negative bacteria following caesarean sections and hysterectomies. Eur J Med Res 4, 126-130.

## Chapter 21

1    Boudana, D., Wolber, A., Coeugniet, E., Martinot-Duquennoy, V., and Pellerin, P. (2010). Une histoire de peau [A history of skin graft]. Annales de Chirurgie Plastique Esthétique *55*, 328-332.

2    Habal, M.B., and Himmel, H.N. (1999). Key issues in plastic and cosmetic surgery (Basel, New York: Karger), pp. 169.

3    Boudana, D., Wolber, A., Coeugniet, E., Martinot-Duquennoy, V., and Pellerin, P. (2010). Une histoire de peau [A history of skin graft]. Annales de Chirurgie Plastique Esthétique *55*, 328-332.

4    Misirlioglu, A., Eroglu, S., Karacaoglan, N., Akan, M., Akoz, T., and Yildirim, S. (2003). Use of honey as an adjunct in the healing of split-thickness skin graft donor site. Dermatol Surg *29*, 168-172.

5    Case history reconstructed from published report and an interview with Cheryl Dunford.

6    Quotes by Jem were published as part of his case history: Dunford, C., Cooper, R., and Molan, P.C. (2000). Using honey as a dressing for infected skin lesions. Nurs Times *96*, 7-9.

7    Traynor, K. (2011). Interview with registered nurse Cheryl Dunford.

8    Ibid.

9    Dunford, C. (2005). The use of honey in wound management. In Honey: A modern wound management product, R. White, R. Cooper, and P. Molan, eds. (Aberdeen, UK: Wounds UK Publishing), pp. 116-129.

10   Ibid.

## Chapter 22

1    American Burn Association (2010). National Burn Repository: Report of Data from 2000-2009.

2    McInnes, M., McInnes, S., and Stanfield, M. (2007). The Hibernation Diet (Souvenier Press).

3    American Burn Association (2010). National Burn Repository: Report of Data from 2000-2009.

4    Malik, K.I., Malik, M.A., and Aslam, A. (2010). Honey compared with silver sulphadiazine in the treatment of superficial partial-thickness burns. Int Wound J *7*, 413-417.

5    American Burn Association (2010). National Burn Repository: Report of Data from 2000-2009.

6    Milenkovic, M., Russo, C.A., and Elixhauser, A. (2007). Hospital Stays for Burns, 2004;  HCUP Statistical Brief #25, Agency for Healthcare Research and Quality, ed. (Rockville, MD).

7    Ebbell, B. (1937). The Papyrus Ebers, the greatest Egyptian medical document (Copenhagen, London,: Levin & Munksgaard; H. Milford, Oxford university

press).

8    Crane, E. (1980). A Book of Honey (Oxford: Oxford University Press). pp. 97

9    Costa-Neto, E.M., and Oliveira, M.V.M. (2000). Cockroach is Good for Asthma: Zootherapeutic Practices in Northeastern Brazil. Research in Human Ecology *7*, 41-51.

10   Blakeney, M. (1999). What is Traditional Knowledge? Why Should it be Protected? Who Should Protect it? For Whom?: Understanding the Value Chain., World Intellectual Property Organization, ed. (Geneva).

11   American Burn Association (2010). National Burn Repository: Report of Data from 2000-2009.

12   Milenkovic, M., Russo, C.A., and Elixhauser, A. (2007). Hospital Stays for Burns, 2004; HCUP Statistical Brief #25, Agency for Healthcare Research and Quality, ed. (Rockville, MD).

13   National Institute of Health (2006). Fact Sheet: Burns and Traumatic Injury, Department of Health and Human Services, ed.

14   American Burn Association (2010). National Burn Repository: Report of Data from 2000-2009.

15   Ibid.

16   Subrahmanyam, M. (1991). Topical application of honey in treatment of burns. Br J Surg *78*, 497-498.

17   Molan, P.C. (2001). Potential of honey in the treatment of wounds and burns. Am J Clin Dermatol *2*, 13-19.

18   Kaufman, T., Eichenlaub, E.H., Angel, M.F., Levin, M., and Futrell, J.W. (1985). Topical acidification promotes healing of experimental deep partial thickness skin burns: a randomised double-blind preliminary study. Burns *12*, 84-90.

19   Subrahmanyam, M. (1993b). Storage of skin grafts in honey. Lancet *341*, 63-64.

20   Ibid.

21   Subrahmanyam, M. (1999). Early tangential excision and skin grafting of moderate burns is superior to honey dressing: a prospective randomised trail. Burns *25*, 729-731.

22   Postmes, T.J., Bosch, M.M.C., Dutrieux, R., van Baare, J., and Hoekstra, M.J. (1997). Speeding up the healing of burns with honey. An experimental study with histological assessment of wound biopsies. In Bee Products: Properties, Applications and Apitherapy, A. Mizrahi, and Y. Lensky, eds. (New York: Plenum Press), pp. 27-37.

23   Kabala-Dzik, A., Stojko, R., Szaflarska-Stojko, E., Wróblewska-Adamek, I., Stojko, A., Stojko, J., and Stawiarska-Pięta, B. (2004). Influence of honey-balm on the rate of scare formation during experimental burn wound healing in pigs. Bull Vet Inst Pulawy *48*, 311-316.

24   Miri, M.R., Hemmati, H., and Shahraki, S. (2005). Comparison of efficacy of

honey versus silver sulfadiazine and acetate mafenid in the treatment of burn wounds in piggies. Pak J Med Sci *21*, 168-173.

25  Subrahmanyam, M. (1998). A prospective randomised clinical and histological study of superficial burn wound healing with honey and silver sulfadiazine. Burns *24*, 157-161.

26  Ibid.

27  Subrahmanyam, M. (1993a). Honey impregnated gauze versus polyurethane film (OpSite*) in the treatment of burns – a prospective randomised study. Br J Plast Surg *46*, 322-323.

28  Subrahmanyam, M. (1994). Honey-impregnated gauze versus amniotic membrane in the treatment of burns. Burns *20*, 331-333.

29  Subrahmanyam, N. (1996b). Addition of antioxidants and polyethylene glycol 4000 enhances the healing property of honey in burns. Ann Burns Fire Disasters *9*, 93-95.

30  Subrahmanyam, M. (1996a). Honey dressing versus boiled potato peel in the treatment of burns: a prospective randomized study. Burns *22*, 491-493.

31  Malik, K.I., Malik, M.A., and Aslam, A. (2010). Honey compared with silver sulphadiazine in the treatment of superficial partial-thickness burns. Int Wound J *7*, 413-417.

32  Hermans, M.H. (1998). Results of a survey on the use of different treatment options for partial and full thickness burns. Burns *24*, 539-551.

33  Bangroo, A.K., Katri, R., and Chauhan, S. (2005). Honey dressing in pediatric burns. J Indian Assoc Pediatr Surg *10*, 172-175.

34  Cooper, R.A., Halas, E., and Molan, P.C. (2002). The efficacy of honey in inhibiting strains of *Pseudomonas aeruginosa* from infected burns. J Burn Care Rehabil *23*, 366-370.

35  Ibid.

36  Henriques, A.F., Jenkins, R.E., Burton, N.F., and Cooper, R.A. (2011). The effect of manuka honey on the structure of Pseudomonas aeruginosa. European Journal of Clininical Microbiology & Infectious Disease *30*, 167-171.

37  Bangroo, A.K., Katri, R., and Chauhan, S. (2005). Honey dressing in pediatric burns. J Indian Assoc Pediatr Surg *10*, 172-175.

38  American Burn Association (2010). National Burn Repository: Report of Data from 2000-2009.

39  Bangroo, A.K., Katri, R., and Chauhan, S. (2005). Honey dressing in pediatric burns. J Indian Assoc Pediatr Surg *10*, 172-175.

40  Mashhood, A.A., Khan, T.A., and Sami, A.N. (2006). Honey compared with 1% silver sulfadiazine cream in the treatment of superficial and partial thickness burns. Journal of Pakistan Association of Dermatologists *16*, 14-19.

41  Grover, S.K., and Prasad, G.C. (1985). Uses of Madhu in ayurveda. J NIMA *10*, 7-10.

42  de Gracia, C.G. (2001). An open study comparing topical silver sulfadiazine

and topical silver sulfadiazine-cerium nitrate in the treatment of moderate and severe burns. Burns *27*, 67-74.

43  Ibid. pp. 72.

44  White, R., and Cutting, K. (2006). Exploring the Effects of Silver in Wound Management. Wounds *18*, 3-7-314.

45  Ibid.

46  Ibid.

47  Ibid.

48  Chung, J.Y., and Herbert, M.E. (2001). Myth: silver sulfadiazine is the best treatment for minor burns. West J Med *175*, 205-206.

49  Subrahmanyam, M. (1998). A prospective randomised clinical and histological study of superficial burn wound healing with honey and silver sulfadiazine. Burns *24*, 157-161.

50  Nagane, N.S., Ganu, J.V., Bhagwat, V.R., and Subramanium, M. (2004). Efficacy of topical honey therapy against silver sulphadiazine treatment in burns: A biochemical study. Indian J Clin Biochem *19*, 173-176.

51  Bangroo, A.K., Katri, R., and Chauhan, S. (2005). Honey dressing in pediatric burns. J Indian Assoc Pediatr Surg *10*, 172-175.

52  Malik, K.I., Malik, M.A., and Aslam, A. (2010). Honey compared with silver sulphadiazine in the treatment of superficial partial-thickness burns. Int Wound J *7*, 413-417.

53  Mashhood, A.A., Khan, T.A., and Sami, A.N. (2006). Honey compared with 1% silver sulfadiazine cream in the treatment of superficial and partial thickness burns. Journal of Pakistan Association of Dermatologists *16*, 14-19.

54  Subrahmanyam, M. (1991). Topical application of honey in treatment of burns. Br J Surg *78*, 497-498.

55  Ibid.


## CHAPTER 23

1  Haas, L.F. (1998). Jean Alfred Fournier (1832-1914). J Neurol Neurosurg Psychiatry 65, 373.

2  Eke, N. (2000). Fournier's gangrene: a review of 1726 cases. Br J Surg 87, 718-728.

3  Ibid.

4  Ibid.

5  Ibid.

6  Smith, G.L., Bunker, C.B., and Dinneen, M.D. (1998). Fournier's gangrene. Br J Urol 81, 347-355.

7  Eke, N. (2000). Fournier's gangrene: a review of 1726 cases. Br J Surg 87, 718-728.

8  Smith, G.L., Bunker, C.B., and Dinneen, M.D. (1998). Fournier's gangrene.

Br J Urol 81, 347-355.

9    Eke, N. (2000). Fournier's gangrene: a review of 1726 cases. Br J Surg 87, 718-728.

10   Smith, G.L., Bunker, C.B., and Dinneen, M.D. (1998). Fournier's gangrene. Br J Urol 81, 347-355.

11   Eke, N. (2000). Fournier's gangrene: a review of 1726 cases. Br J Surg 87, 718-728.

12   Smith, G.L., Bunker, C.B., and Dinneen, M.D. (1998). Fournier's gangrene. Br J Urol 81, 347-355. P 352

13   Leaper, D.J. (1992). Eusol. BMJ 304, 930-931.

14   Patton, M.A. Ibid.Eusol: the continuing controversy. 1636.

15   Efem, S.E.E. (1993). Recent advances in the management of Fournier's gangrene: Preliminary observations. Surgery 113, 200-204.

16   Ibid.

17   Ibid.

18   Hejase, M.J., Simonin, J.E., Bihrle, R., and Coogan, C.L. (1996). Genital Fournier's gangrene: experience with 38 patients. Urology 47, 734-739.

19   Ibid.

20   Ibid.

## CHAPTER 24

1    Ingle, R., Levin, J., and Polinder, K. (2006). Wound healing with honey - a randomised controlled trial. S Afr Med J 96, 831-835.

2    Ibid.

## INTERLUDE 9

1    Ransome, H.M. (1937). The Sacred Bee in Ancient Times and Folklore (London: George Allen and Unwin).

2    Budge, E.A.W. (1896). The Life and Exploits of Alexander the Great (London: Cambridge University Press). pp. 349.

3    Ibid. pp. 376.

## PART IV
## CHAPTER 25

1    Liss, M. (2008). Interview of Michael Liss, a homeopathic consultant and certified naturopathic doctor in Frederick County, MD, K. Traynor, ed. (Frederick, MD).

2    Palmer, L. (2007). California Sea Lion Receives Sweet Treatment After Shark Attack. Am Bee J 147, 273-274.

3   Puotinen, C. (2007). A honey of a cure: all the products made by bees have special gifts for dogs. In Whole Dog Journal.

4   National Honey Board (2005). Going to the Dogs. In The Nucleus (Longmont, CO: National Honey Board), pp. 6.

5   Zacharias, M. (2008). Natural Rearing of Dogs.

6   Department of Animal Science. Mastitis in Dairy Cows (Macdonald Campus of McGill University, Faculty of Agricultural & Environmental Sciences).

7   Allen, K.L., and Molan, P.C. (1997). The sensitivity of mastitis-causing bacteria to the antibacterial activity of honey. N Z J Agric Res 40, 537-540.

8   Fennell, C. (1979). The treatment of teat lesions in milking cows with a pollen extract creams - a clinical trial. Ir Vet J 33, 151-155.